T0355054

PRAISE FOR
THE BIG 100

"More and more people are living for 100 years—or longer. William J. Kole uses his knowledge and personal experiences to suggest how we can use these bonus years to best advantage, for ourselves and others. With beautiful prose and a sense of fun, *The Big 100* is stimulating and inspiring. You should definitely read it."

—**Dr. Jane Goodall**, founder of
the Jane Goodall Institute and UN Messenger of Peace

"*The Big 100* is an entertaining challenge to all of us to rethink the second half of our lives. Provocative and fun."

—**Dr. John Beard**, director,
International Longevity Center-USA

"William J. Kole is more than a brilliant journalist and dazzling storyteller. He is a time traveler. Kole is our guide to a coming world of super-longevity and what it means for health systems, policy makers, and the very fabric of families and communities. *The Big 100* is our future. There is no more compelling story."

—**Brian Murphy**, author of
*81 Days Below Zero: The Incredible Survival Story
of a World War II Pilot in Alaska's Frozen Wilderness*

"With rapidly aging populations across the world and longer lives ahead, William J. Kole's *The Big 100* could not have come at a more important time. It's a compelling call to action for everyone interested in the challenges and opportunities of our great demographic shift and the potential for longer, healthier, and more fulfilling lives."

—**Paul Irving**, founding chair of
the Milken Institute's Center for the Future of Aging
and distinguished scholar-in-residence at the University of
Southern California's Leonard Davis School of Gerontology

"Optimizing human longevity was arguably the greatest achievement of the last century, thanks in great part to the successes of public health. Enabling healthy longevity and the assets that older people contribute to the world will be our all-of-society challenge for the current generation. William J. Kole's book gives us a basis for envisioning the society we want to design for all of our longer lives as we each approach 'The Big 100.'"

—**Dr. Linda P. Fried**, dean of
Columbia University's Mailman School of Public Health
and director of the Robert N. Butler Columbia Aging Center

"Do I want to live to 100? I don't know. But I do know that in *The Big 100*, journalist William J. Kole makes me think about it with a newfound appreciation for the science of aging. I had never truly considered the enormous societal cost of people living longer until *The Big 100*. Centenarians are the fastest-growing segment of our population, and Kole forces us to ask if we are ready for that tectonic demographic shift. Kole provides valuable perspective around the science of aging, the impact on society as people reach that milestone, and some heartwarming personal touches."

—**Doug Most**, bestselling author of
*The Race Underground: Boston, New York, and
the Incredible Rivalry that Built America's First Subway*

"None of us knows whether we'll make it to 'The Big 100,' but regardless of age, all of us should make sure we have a copy of William J. Kole's book on our shelf! In a readable style and an easy voice, Kole uses hard data and personal stories to explore everything important about the aging journey—finances, health, work, diet, dignity, laughter, and love. *The Big 100* tells the most human story in the most human terms."

—**Stephen Puleo**, author of
Dark Tide, *The Caning*, and *Voyage of Mercy*

"*The Big 100* points the way to a great long life without minimizing pain or the emotional weight of mortality. Using the latest scientific evidence for optimism and telling inspiring, sometimes amusing, stories of people as old as a hundred and more, William J. Kole shows how you can find joy in life right up to your last days on earth."

—**Francine Russo**, bestselling author of
Love After 50: How to Find It, Enjoy It, and Keep It

"Many people say they want to live to be a hundred, but beyond pension plans and good insurance, there's not really much of a road map for getting the most from that incredible milestone. William J. Kole's cogent exploration of 'super-agers' is a blueprint for living your best life long after most people are preparing to check out. I'm truly energized about my golden years in ways I wouldn't have thought possible."

—**Rachel Jones**,
National Press Foundation

"Deeply researched and reported, written in brisk, sharp prose, William J. Kole's probing exploration of the implications of longevity and an ever-expanding lifespan is a compelling and vital read. It's a timely and fascinating analysis of the cultural, economic, racial, medical, philosophical, societal, and political upsides and downsides of the coming global surge in the number of centenarians. It's also great storytelling and a provocative look ahead at what the future of aging means for us all."

—**Neal Thompson**, author of
The First Kennedys: The Humble Roots of an
American Dynasty and *A Curious Man: The Strange*
& Brilliant Life of Robert "Believe It or Not" Ripley

THE BIG
100

UNCOVERING THE KEYS TO
LONGEVITY

WILLIAM J. KOLE

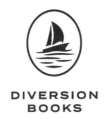

DIVERSION
BOOKS

For Terry.
I love growing older with you.

Published by Diversion Books
Book design by Neuwirth & Associates, Inc.

Have You Done What You Wanted to Do
Copyright © 2022 by Peter Prengaman, used with permission of the author.

First Diversion Books Hardcover Edition, October 2023
First Diversion Books Trade Paperback Edition, December 2024
Hardcover ISBN 978-1-6357-6856-5
Trade Paperback ISBN 978-1-63576-992-0
e-ISBN 978-1-6357-6999-9

Printed in the United States of America
1 3 5 7 9 10 8 6 4 2

CONTENTS

MERELY ONE HUNDRED
AND ONE

It's 2050 in Boston and, in the self-proclaimed Hub of the Universe, some things never change. The traffic is satanic, the Red Sox are breaking hearts, and the biotech sector has gone from boom to bust to boom again. None of that, though, explains the scene playing out on eternally elegant Newbury Street:

A well-dressed, impeccably coiffed woman leans over a glass counter at Cartier, sparring with a salesperson over her senior discount for the emerald- and onyx-encrusted panther brooch shimmering on a rectangle of black velvet. Fit, energetic, and spray-tanned, the elderly customer extends the inside of her wrist to the clerk, who uses a wand to scan the tiny tattoos containing her driver's license, credit cards, and AARP membership profile.

Her profile pops up on a 3D hologram screen in the air between them, and the clerk raises an eyebrow.

"I do apologize, madam," she tells the customer, "but I'm afraid you're only entitled to a discount if you're 105. Store policy."

Merely 101, the indignant client slings her Valentino silk scarf over her shoulder, pivots on one high heel, and stalks out of the shop without another word, leaving behind only staccato clicks on Cartier's white marble floor.

AN OUTLANDISH SCENARIO? MAYBE NOT. SIXTY-FIVE, THE TRADI-tional age to cash in on a senior discount, hasn't been "old" for a long time now. Our societies are graying at an unprecedented rate and in unparalleled ways. Someday soon, we may find ourselves living in a world in which turning sixty-five could mean we're only half done.

One hundred and one, a remarkable life span today, may not be so exceptional tomorrow. What follows is our journey to this threshold and the super-aging world beyond, and with it, a hard examination of what we must do now to ensure our longer lives will truly be worth living.

CHAPTER ONE

A WRINKLE IN TIME

It arrived the other day, sandwiched between the gas bill and a local politician's plea for campaign contributions, and concealed within a red-and-white envelope. It looked innocuous enough. But as I tore open the sleeve to reveal the contents, a sense of dread washed over me.

Anthrax? A kidnapper's ransom note? An income tax audit? None of the above, but somehow, this felt worse. It was an AARP card. With *my* name on it.

"What the hell am I supposed to do with this? I'm only sixty-one, for God's sake," I muttered to myself, crumpling the envelope and striding toward our kitchen garbage can. I trashed the accompanying letter, but, almost as an afterthought, I kept the plastic card—not primarily because it promised senior discounts for select goods and services, but because it was stout and sturdy, perfect for scraping ice off my car windshield during our interminable New England winters.

Don't judge me. You'll be in your early sixties someday, too, if you're not already there—or older, with all the attendant denial and dismay, gray (or, in my case, no) hair, and chronic backaches. I mean absolutely no disrespect to AARP (formerly known as the American Association of Retired Persons), which does noble and supremely important work. It's just that AARP cards and senior discounts and access to restaurants' early bird specials are startling reminders that I'm growing older. And in this, I suspect, I am not alone. Our attitude toward aging, if expressed as a relationship status: It's complicated.

If it's any consolation (it is to me), less than a century ago, sixty-one would have been an age to die for.

In the late 1920s, it was the average American's life expectancy at birth. But sixty-one also has a unique and mystical resonance for me, because it marks precisely the halfway point of the longest verifiable human lifetime there ever was—a life that briefly and improbably intersected with my own.

So, sit back and relax; pour yourself a glass of milk, Merlot, or Metamucil; and allow me to tell you the story of that extraordinary life. Because in the not-so-distant future, our encounters with super-agers are going to become routine. And some of us—many more of us, in fact, than you might imagine—are destined to find them gazing back at us, quizzically, in the mirror.

SHE WAS, IN THE END, AN ACCIDENTAL QUEEN.

Blind now, and nearly deaf, she waved regally from a turquoise wheelchair as an attendant pushed her out to meet the press. This monarch's royalty was rooted in a quirk of biology, and her coat of arms was DNA's signature double helix, but none of that diminished her celebrity. Why should it? Fifteen minutes of fame was the least that was due to a woman who'd rightfully been dubbed *la doyenne de l'humanité.*

News photographers jockeyed for position and camera motor drives whirred and clicked as she was wheeled into place. Then the room fell silent. All eyes peered intently into hers, enigmatic and clouded by cataracts. A doctor knelt at her side, cupping his hands to shout a question into her right ear, but the loss of her hearing and sight hardly mattered. The media had come because of all she *had* seen, heard, and experienced so unfathomably long ago.

A brief but unmistakable twinkle glimmered in the sheen of her ancient eyes, and the faintest of smirks enlivened a face creased with wrinkles. And then Jeanne Calment began to hold forth. She was 121. I was thirty-five, a newly minted foreign correspondent in France for the Associated Press. And I was instantly smitten.

I was also panged with guilt: It was my wife's thirty-ninth birthday, and I was anxious to hop an early train back to our home in the leafy Paris suburb of Noisy-le-Roi, so I could properly celebrate the conclusion of her fourth decade around the sun with our eight-year-old son and five-year-old daughter. But let's face it: It's not every day that one gets a chance to write about the oldest person on the planet. And as Calment began to speak, it was clear that I wouldn't regret lingering.

"I only have one wrinkle and I'm sitting on it," she said, flirting with the reporters like a woman a quarter of her age. It was a year before her death at 122 years and 164 days, and we'd assembled for a most improbable news conference: She was releasing a four-track rap CD titled *Time's Mistress*, hip-hopping to a musical genre fully a century younger than she was.

By now, she'd given up her most beloved vices: two lightly puffed cigarettes a day and a single glass of port wine before meals. Even so, she regaled the spellbound scrum of international journalists, vividly recalling her travels to Paris as a young girl while the Eiffel Tower was still under construction. She reminisced about working in her father's art supply store in the southern French city of Arles, selling colored pencils to Vincent van Gogh in 1888 when he was experimenting with Impressionism "and still had his ear." She said van Gogh was ugly as sin and reeked of absinthe: "We called him 'Le Dingo.'"

Her long life was at once ordinary and extraordinary.

She was born on February 21, 1875, just four years after France lost the Franco-Prussian War; ten years after Abraham Lincoln was assassinated; and a year before Alexander Graham Bell invented the telephone. She was twenty when moving pictures were invented; nearly forty at the start of World War I; already retired when Germany invaded France at the start of World War II; and lived through the administrations of twenty-seven French presidents. Her last, Jacques Chirac, would say of her passing: "She was a little bit the grandmother of all of us."

She dabbled in painting and piano, but never had what could be described as a proper profession. She took fencing lessons at age eighty-five and didn't stop riding her bicycle until she turned 100. For years thereafter, she lived a disciplined, almost ascetic life, rising at 6:45 a.m. to start each day with prayers and calisthenics.

In 1965, when Madame Calment turned ninety, her notary public, forty-seven-year-old lawyer André-François Raffray, approached her with what he was certain was a very shrewd play for her apartment on the posh Rue Gambetta in central Arles. Raffray invoked en viager, an ancient French arrangement in which a buyer pays an older owner a lump sum for the property and further agrees to pay a certain amount every month until the owner dies.

The lawyer must have rubbed his hands together in glee and self-congratulation at the bargain before him. It was a sweetheart deal; the con of a lifetime. Just not Raffray's. He died thirty years later, at age seventy, after having paid Calment more than double what the apartment was worth—something to the tune of $200,000— without ever having lived there himself. Had he done his homework, Monsieur Raffray might have known he was tempting fate: Calment's father lived to ninety-four, and an unusually high number of her ancestors lived deep into their seventies in the 1600s and 1700s, an era when forty was a ripe old age.

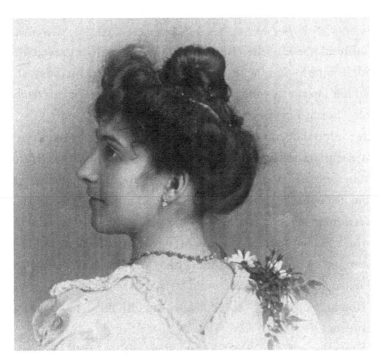

Jeanne Calment at age twenty. She lived to 122 years and 164 days. (*Sipa/Rex/ Shutterstock via Creative Commons/OpenVerse*)

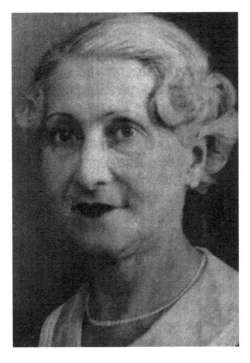

Jeanne Calment at seventy, with another half a century yet to go. (*Paris Match via Creative Commons/OpenVerse*)

Calment was 120 when they buried the lawyer. The gravediggers wouldn't come for her for another two years. On every birthday, she'd teased her lawyer by sending a card that read: *Désolé, je suis toujours vivante.* "Sorry, I'm still alive."

Her only public comment after Raffray's death was shy and wry—the quintessential Gallic shrug: "In life, one sometimes makes bad deals."

At her 120th birthday bash, blurting, "Why all the applause?" she was pushed with great fanfare in her wheelchair across a floor strewn with red roses to her favorite meal—a spread so incredibly indulgent, one wonders how on earth she ever managed to live so long if this was her comfort food. Too many dinners like this—foie gras, duck thighs, cheese, and chocolate cake—would do in most mortals.

"How are you doing?" asked France's health minister, one of 300 VIP guests.

"Everything's fine," she responded, feeble and frail but impeccably coiffed and stylishly dressed in black and white.

Seven months and twenty-two days later, Calment would surpass Shigechiyo Izumi—a Japanese man who died in 1986—as the oldest person of all time with a verifiable birth date, a title she still holds today. Asked to describe her vision of the future, she replied impishly: "Very brief." She was, she said, "waiting for death and the journalists."

Hilarity, like longevity, was one of her strong suits.

Along with genetics.

BRACE FOR A TECTONIC SHIFT IN EARTH'S DEMOGRAPHICS OVER THE next few decades.

More of us than ever before in human history are achieving the exceptional age of 100, 105, 110, or even older. "All societies in the world are in the midst of this longevity revolution," the United Nations cautions in a little-noticed but no less remarkable report.

"Some are at its early stages and some are more advanced. But all will pass through this extraordinary transition."

None of this should come as a surprise. Doctors have been telling us that living to and beyond 100 is simply the result of better control over the risk factors for heart disease and stroke along with significant dents in cancer mortality. But we're aging in numbers never before imagined. In the United States, Europe, Japan, and elsewhere, it's a rapidly unfolding yet largely unnoticed phenomenon that's catching health care and Social Security policymakers, financial planning specialists, and ordinary families off guard. The coronavirus pandemic and the nationwide opioids crisis, which reduced life expectancy, are expected to be temporary setbacks on our collective march to 100.

We're already seeing the clouds gather on the horizon. The trust funds that support Social Security are projected to run out of money by the mid-2030s—coinciding exactly with when the centenarian surge will begin to crest. And already, elder care is busting Medicare and Medicaid budgets.

Social Security was designed when people lived only a few years after retiring. What happens when sixty-five is merely a life half-lived?

"Look, we're facing a retirement crunch that's only going to get worse," says US senator Elizabeth Warren of Massachusetts, who's been pushing for a major increase in monthly benefits beyond those periodic cost-of-living adjustments. "Social Security has kept millions of older Americans out of poverty. Most retirees rely on it. It's money for prescriptions, money for gas, money for food, money for a trip to see the grandkids. Without action, future generations are likely to be even worse off."

Exceptional aging is all about numbers, so let's consider what they're telling us about this coming demographic shift.

The year 2030, the US Census Bureau says, will mark what it terms "a demographic turning point" for the United States. We define the baby boom generation as encompassing those born between 1946 and 1964, and in the world of demography, that group is hugely influential. Already, one in five Americans is a boomer, and in 2030, they'll all be older than sixty-five, the traditional retirement age in the minds of the minions. Just four years later, in 2034, older adults (those aged sixty-five and beyond) will outnumber children (those aged seventeen and younger) for the first time in US history.

And more than aging boomers is powering this lurch in extreme longevity. Effective new ways to combat cancer, heart attack, and stroke are vastly improving the outlook for our youngest humans: those who comprise Generations Alpha and Beta. Astonishing new research by the Stanford Center on Longevity (at Stanford University) says fully half of today's American five-year-olds can expect to reach 100—a life span experts there think will become the norm for newborns by 2050. "The New Map of Life," SCL calls it, noting that our kids and grandkids are going to live through "one of the most profound transformations of the human experience."

I've got a five-year-old grandson. Is he a centenarian in the making? It's a thought I can't shake every time I watch him kick a soccer ball in our backyard or seamlessly navigate his Nintendo Switch on our living room sofa.

Those who've hit 100 often scarcely can believe it themselves. Among America's newly minted centenarians was Norman Lear, the Emmy Award–winning television producer and cofounder of the advocacy organization People for the American Way, who died in 2023. In a guest essay for the *New York Times* published on his 100th birthday, the man famed for producing iconic TV shows, including *All in the Family, Maude, The Jeffersons,* and *Good Times,* wrote: "Well, I made it. I am 100 years old today. I wake up every morning grateful to be alive."

"It is remarkable to consider that television—the medium for which I am most well-known—did not even exist when I was born, in 1922," he marveled.

But with the promise of those extra years comes a cautionary note. "It is not enough to reimagine or rethink society to become longevity-ready; we must build it, and fast," the Stanford Center warns.

America's northern neighbor is already experiencing the imbalance of a graying populace. For the first time in Canadian history, there are more seniors than there are children. Centenarians are the single fastest-growing age bracket, and the gap between the ultra-young and über-old continues to widen. "There's no coming back," says Laurent Martel, chief demographer at Statistics Canada.

"It's great that people are living longer," says Jane Philpott, a physician and former Canadian health minister who is now dean of the Queen's University Faculty of Health Sciences. But, she adds: "It does, of course, raise concerns as it relates to the sustainability of our health care system. . . . There's no reason for panic."

Panic? No. But acknowledgment and urgent contemplation? Yes. And purposeful action? Most definitely.

By 2035, the Census Bureau projects, the number of Americans aged eighty-five and older will nearly double to almost 12 million. By 2060, it will more than triple to 19 million. Aging boomers and rising life expectancy will cause the eighty-five-plus crowd to grow by nearly 200 percent over the next four decades. And while all that is happening, the United States alone will add half a million centenarians. In less than three decades, the number of people aged 100 or older is projected to be 3.7 million worldwide. That's equivalent to the current number of people living in Connecticut, or nearly everyone in Los Angeles, hitting 100-plus. By 2100, the United Nations' population division projects, there will be more than 25 million centenarians. And billions more worldwide who don't quite make it to 100 nonetheless will live significantly deeper into their eighties and nineties.

The United States leads the world in the number of centenarians with just under 100,000, followed by Japan, China, and India. By 2050, China and Japan are expected to dominate, but don't count out Europe. Italy isn't far behind Japan in terms of oldest population, followed by Finland, Portugal, and Greece. Southern Europe—specifically, Croatia, Greece, Italy, Malta, Portugal, Serbia, Slovenia, and Spain—has the oldest population on the planet, with the lowest birth rates and the greatest numbers of citizens older than sixty-five.

Japan, the world's grayest nation with nearly one in three people aged sixty-five or older, already is considering action. Little wonder: Japan's Ministry of Health, Labor and Welfare announced late in 2022 that the number of centenarians in the country exceeded 90,000 for the first time, increasing fivefold over the past two decades. The government is looking at reclassifying Japanese in the sixty-five-to-seventy-four bracket as no longer elderly but "pre-old age." Why? The Japan Gerontological Society and the Japan Geriatrics Society check off several reasons: Half of those between sixty-five and seventy-four hold jobs, only 6 percent need help caring for themselves, and studies have shown most even walk as fast as those in their fifties did in decades past.

And Japan was home to a woman with remarkable staying power who came close to becoming the next Jeanne Calment. Born in 1903, Kane Tanaka loved playing the board game Othello and enjoyed studying mathematics right up until her death at 119 in 2022. She long topped the leaderboard in a country that, like clockwork, churns out supercentenarians, defined as anyone who lives to 110 or beyond. The reasons are as numerous as Tanaka's years: Japan's culinary tradition emphasizes fish, rice, vegetables, and other foods low in fat; and age traditionally is revered, so people tend to stay active and feel useful well into their eighties and beyond.

Calment's latest challenger was, appropriately, a fellow Frenchwoman. France has an estimated 21,000 centenarians, the French statistics agency Insee (National Institute of Statistics and Economic Studies) says, and nearly four dozen of them are 110 or older. Lucile Randon, a nun also known as Sister André, knew how to party: She toasted all her birthdays in adulthood with a traditional cocktail of equal parts port and chocolate. But she grew weary of the burdens of age, and the world's oldest living nun and oldest survivor of COVID-19 died early in 2023, just a few weeks shy of her 119th birthday.

The oldest living person in the world was, until her death at age 117 in August, an American-born Spaniard, Maria Branyas Morera. "I am old, very old, but not an idiot," Branyas's cheeky Twitter bio read. She told Guinness World Records she attributed her longevity to "order, tranquility, good connection with family and friends, contact with nature, emotional stability, no worries, no regrets, lots of positivity,

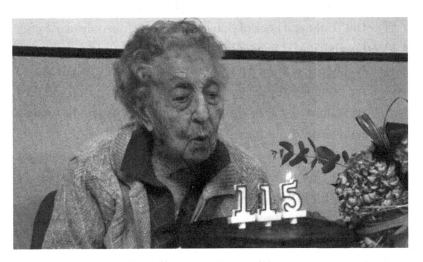

Maria Branyas Morera, the world's oldest living person until her death at 117 in 2024, blows out the candles on her 115th birthday cake. (© *Residència Santa Maria del Tura*)

and staying away from toxic people." Branyas, who lived through the 1918 influenza epidemic, both world wars, and the Spanish Civil War, also survived a bout with COVID-19 at age 113. "I haven't done anything extraordinary," the soft-spoken supercentenarian told the Barcelona newspaper *La Vanguardia*. "The only thing I did was live."

Right behind her are 116-year-old Tomika Itooka of Japan, who at 100 was still climbing the long stone steps to Ashiya Shrine without a cane, and Inah Canabarro Lucas, a 116-year-old Brazilian.

To paraphrase the late Norris McWhirter, founding editor of the *Guinness Book of Records*, as he immortalized Jeanne Calment's longevity: Staying alive is the most competitive of all records. After all, 8 billion of us are at it.

And in the swiftly graying world that awaits us, we're all going to encounter astonishingly old versions of ourselves far more frequently than we do now.

You'd be forgiven if you ever heard someone described as being "as old as Methuselah" and thought to yourself: *Who's that?*

The Old Testament book of Genesis mentions him only in passing, but Methuselah is said to have lived to 969. Apart from his longevity, the biblical figure is known only for his father, Enoch, who's said to have never tasted death because he was so faithful that God whisked him away; and for his far more famous grandson, Noah, the world's best-known boatbuilder (for all the wrong reasons).

Adam, purportedly the first of us all, is said to have lived to 930; Jared (Enoch's father) to 962; and Noah himself to 950. Among Bible literalists, theories persist even now of a scriptural "firmament"—imagined as a sort of ozone-like atmospheric membrane that purportedly kept the Earth moist and tropical while also guarding it from the sun's destructive ultraviolet rays, allowing human life to achieve fantastic proportions until that protective layer gradually faded away, taking our life expectancy with it. Conservative theologians introduce an even-harder-to-quantify element: Generation by generation, our collective sin—expressed in serial wrongdoing, a persistent culture of murderous violence, and willful environmental degradation—steadily chipped away at those once-epic life spans.

Scholars offer a more plausible explanation: Well-intentioned yet bungled translations of scripture mistakenly rendered the original Hebrew word for "month" as a "year." Viewed anew through that lens, suddenly it all makes sense: Methuselah's 969 lunar months become a far more realistic eighty solar years.

And for the skeptics, there's always Genesis 6:3. "My Spirit will not contend with man forever, for he is mortal; his days shall be 120 years," it reads. That, of course, aligns almost perfectly with the glorious arc of Jeanne Calment's life. It's almost as though God himself is winking at us, like a distant star in the heavens.

Meanwhile, Methuselah—the man, the myth, the legend—continues to captivate humankind. His namesake, a 4,854-year-old Great Basin bristlecone pine known as the Methuselah Tree, is still growing strong high in the White Mountains of eastern California. It's the oldest known tree with the greatest confirmed age on Earth—a sort of arboreal equivalent to Madame Calment.

There are modern Methuselahs, supposedly—if we're to believe those supermarket tabloid accounts of individuals alleged to have achieved a fanciful age.

Mbah Gotho was such a person. When he died in 2017, the Indonesian gentleman—known by one name, Sodimejo, as is commonplace in that country—had a plastic identity card indicating he was born on December 31, 1870. That would have made him 146. A farmer, fisherman, and lifelong chain-smoker, his earliest memory was the ceremonial opening of a sugar factory in 1880, when his homeland was under Dutch colonial rule.

He cheated death, as the story goes, in somewhat spectacular fashion: Gotho's family had had his tombstone chiseled in 1992, when he was "only" 122. Allegedly, of course, he had the last laugh, vastly outliving them all. Or maybe it was the last cry: Just months before his death, having outlived all ten of his siblings, all four of his wives, and all his children, he told a reporter: "All I want is to die."

It's a compelling story. There's just one problem: Indonesia didn't start recording births until 1900, throwing the birth date on his laminated ID into serious doubt.

Did Mbah Gotho really live to 146? Maybe. It's not out of the realm of possibility. Photos of his sunken eyes and cheeks and his crepe skin make him look positively ancient. But the proof is in the paper, and on that score, Jeanne Calment has the goods. Calment retains her place in history as the oldest person whose age can be authenticated by official documents—in her case, a municipal birth certificate from Arles dated February 21, 1875, a baptismal record from a Roman Catholic curate dated two days later, and a slew of other church and census paperwork.

Even, and perhaps especially, Madame Calment's claim to fame has been questioned numerous times. It began long before her death

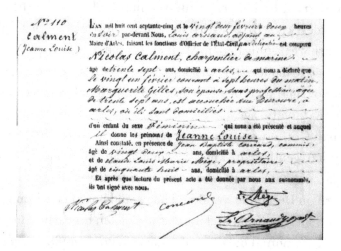

Jeanne Calment's birth certificate. She was born on February 21, 1875. (*City of Arles, France*)

on August 4, 1997, which grabbed headlines until Britain's Princess Diana followed a few weeks later, knocking everything else off the front pages. Challenges to Calment's incredible longevity were inevitable. Yet, in her case, the most recent and strident doubts were demonstrably unscientific—and abruptly laid to rest.

In 2018, Russian gerontologist Valery Novoselov floated a conspiracy theory claiming that Calment died in 1934, and her daughter posed as her mother to avoid paying inheritance taxes. An exhaustive study published in 2019 in the *Journals of Gerontology* debunked that notion, concluding: "Jeanne Calment's claim as the record-holder for longevity for the human species, at 122 years and 164 days, remains valid." Enticingly, the French authors added: "Calment's age can be reached and even exceeded, even though the probability remains very low." They demanded that Novoselov retract his claim. As of this writing, he has yet to do so.

Jean-Marie Robine, a longevity expert with France's National Institute of Health and Medical Research, visited Calment regularly and noted what he called her "extraordinary resistance to sickness, stress, and depression." He found Calment to be a curious case: "There's nothing exceptional about her lifestyle. She's not athletic, not a health fanatic. She says she's interested in everything, but not really passionate about anything."

What's most astonishing is that, since the dawn of time, an estimated 117 billion members of our species have been born on Earth, according to the Population Reference Bureau, a Washington, DC–based nonprofit research group—and Calment is the only one we know for certain who has lived to 122.

She not only survived but thrived. At 121, a year before her death, she was shown how to use a computer and promptly set up her own website. "I dream, I think, I go over my life," she said. "I never get bored."

When she finally made her exit after 44,724 days, hundreds gathered at Arles's church to bid her adieu. The tributes scribbled in a condolence book capture her impact and reach. One, in Japanese, reads: "Bravo to the person who made death wait."

How long will her reign as oldest verified human endure? With the coming surge of centenarians bearing down, it's entirely possible that the next Jeanne Calment has already been born, raised a family, and retired. He, she, or they may even have been given a grim diagnosis, never daring to imagine that the disease threatening to cut their life short is about to be eradicated, throwing open an intoxicating new range of life span possibilities.

Who knows? It might even be you.

FACED WITH THE INEVITABILITY OF COMMONPLACE SUPER-AGING, scientists are focusing more on extending our health spans (the period of life spent in good health) to match our lengthening life spans. Can we have it both ways? If the answer is no, what's the point of living triple-digit lives when our final decades are going to be spent battling chronic and debilitating illness?

"You don't want to live to be over 100 years old if the last twenty years of your life are spent in pain and sickness," S. Jay Olshansky, an epidemiologist and longevity expert at the University of Illinois at Chicago, writes in the *Journal of the American Medical Association*. "Ideally, you want to compress the years of decay and disease—what I call the 'red zone'—into as few as possible at the very end of life. We should not continue to pursue life extension without considering the health consequences of living longer lives."

All of this prompts a much more immediate question: What happens when we all live to 100, or when most of us at least come close? It's tempting to brush that aside, but we do so at our peril.

If we don't start preparing today, we'll pay a horrible price. Men and women routinely will have to work deep into their seventies and eighties. Elderly poverty rates will soar as centenarians vastly outlive their savings. Social isolation and suicide will stain society as never before. Younger generations who've traditionally depended on inheritances to buy a home or pay for their own kids' higher education will be left empty-handed. And those of us who end up living deep into our 100s may outlast our spouses and children, depriving us of loving care.

Who will take care of us? Home health and personal care aides are among the fastest-growing occupations in the United States, according to the Bureau of Labor Statistics, which forecasts 1.2 million new such jobs between now and 2026. But most Americans don't want to bathe or otherwise care for the elderly. Little wonder that annual staffing turnover in nursing homes approaches a staggering 75 percent.

Immigrants traditionally have filled the gap. Massachusetts, where I grew up, is home to America's third-largest Haitian expatriate community after Florida and New York, and skilled and compassionate Haitian nurses capably dominate the state's home-health-care niche. Poles, Slovaks, and other central and eastern Europeans do the same on that continent. "There is actually no way to meet the demands of care without a strong immigrant workforce," says Ai-jen Poo, president of the National Domestic Workers Alliance and executive director of a caregiver network called Caring Across Generations. Long-term, though, relying on immigrant caregivers may not be sustainable, given the fraught and highly charged political debate around immigration in both the United States and Europe. And in this country, it's even more complicated: Medicare doesn't pay for long-term care unless medical attention is needed.

Don't underestimate any of this, warns Chris Farrell, an expert on the economics of extreme aging. "Centenarians are rapidly moving from society's fringes into the mainstream," he says. "This longevity transformation is a clarion call for the nation to take the economics of an aging population seriously. Without major policy changes by the US government and employers, a future with swelling numbers of octogenarians, nonagenarians, and centenarians is potentially grim."

Some nations, notably Japan and the United Kingdom, have awakened to the devastating effects of social isolation on aging societies: The governments of both have added "ministers of loneliness" to their cabinets. It makes sense, says Eddy Elmer, a Dutch-Canadian gerontology researcher. Chronic loneliness, he says, "causes a wear and tear on the body that becomes more pronounced over time."

It's only in its infancy, but the specter of living decades beyond our wildest imaginations, lonely, and broke, is spawning a new niche in the retirement planning industry: longevity coaching. Similar to life coaches who've long helped us set goals and achieve dreams, longevity coaches work with us not only to make beneficial lifestyle choices but to prepare us financially so we don't outlive our money.

Extreme longevity also is destined to complicate how we're collectively walking the blood- and tear-stained path toward a meaningful reckoning of racial injustice—and not just in the United States, but globally. Setting aside Asia, eight in ten of the world's centenarians are white, making the realm of 100 and older a hostile environment for Black and brown people.

SCIENTISTS DIGGING INTO WHY THIS IS THE CASE INCREASINGLY are coalescing around "weathering"—the theory that systemic racism, resulting in a statistically greater exposure to violence, poorer nutrition, and higher incidences of diabetes and heart disease, takes a cumulative toll on Blacks, Latinos, and Native Americans, putting them at a distinct disadvantage when it comes to achieving exceptional ages. Although inheriting the right genes is the single biggest driver of extreme longevity, there *are* other factors: eating cleanly, exercising regularly, and enjoying a solid socioeconomic status at midlife. And for much of the world, those things are out of reach.

Arline Geronimus, a University of Michigan public health and population researcher who coined the term "weathering" and has done pioneering work on the subject, says the practical effects of entrenched racism start early in life.

"Marginalized Americans are disproportionately more likely to suffer from chronic diseases and to die at much younger ages than their middle- and upper-class white counterparts," she says in a newly published study. "Systemic injustice—not just in the form of racist cops but in the form of everyday life—takes a physical, too often deadly toll on Black, Brown, poor, and other culturally oppressed and politically marginalized communities." (Much more on this alarming phenomenon in chapter 4.)

As our planet ages, ageism—discrimination based on a person's age, whether old or young—is sharply increasing. In its 2021 global report on ageism, the United Nations says health care rationing on the basis of age is widespread. Worldwide, the United Nations warns, one in two people are ageist against older people, and in Europe, the only region where data is available, one in three elderly citizens say they've been a target of ageism.

In his bestselling novel *Boomsday,* Christopher Buckley introduces us to Cassandra Devine, a charismatic twenty-nine-year-old blogger who's deeply disturbed by the baby boomers' huge drain on Social Security. Her indecent proposal: Give boomers government incentives to agree to be euthanized, or "transitioned," before they turn seventy-five. Cultural warfare predictably erupts as a US senator with presidential ambitions campaigns on the idea.

Fast-forward to today, and Buckley's fictitious Absurdistan doesn't seem nearly as far-fetched as it did in 2007.

Consider Yusuke Narita, an assistant professor of economics in his late thirties at Yale, who has repeatedly and publicly suggested a shocking combination of mass suicide and euthanasia as the "only solution" to the societal burdens of rapid aging in his native Japan. Narita, who insists he's misunderstood, has been roundly condemned. But there's no doubt that millennials and members of Generation Z have a problem with boomers. Angered by many of that generation's perceived affinity for Trump-style, political arch-conservatism, ambivalence toward climate change, affinity for guns, and smug assurance of pensions and other sources of wealth that seem destined to die with them, the younger sets have coined the condescending term, "Okay boomer."

Imagine their dismay as centenarians form the vanguard of a vast shuffling corps of elders who drain public resources and exert outsized influence on virtually every facet of modern life. (Spoiler alert: It's already happening. People aged sixty-five and up are the biggest voting bloc in most states. By 2040, the senior population is projected to swell by 44 percent, while the eighteen-to-sixty-four population grows by just 6 percent.)

"Older politicians have an advantage at the polls because their fellow older citizens are much more likely to cast a ballot than the young," Thomas Klassen, a professor of public policy at Canada's York University, writes in a commentary for *The Conversation*. Historically in US presidential elections, he notes, more than 70 percent of voters aged sixty and older cast ballots, compared to fewer than 50 percent of those aged eighteen to twenty-nine.

That's an admittedly dystopian vision of our rapidly graying planet's future. Unfortunately, it's an entirely plausible outcome if we ignore the transformative changes our coming age of extreme longevity will bring about. But if we get this right, there's ample reason for optimism and hope.

HITTING 100 IS A BIG DEAL, BUT IT NO LONGER AUTOMATICALLY triggers newspaper headlines or draws the local television news crew to the retirement home, if only because there's already so many of these venerable souls.

That's understandable. It's also regrettable. Exceptionally long life doesn't automatically equate to exceptional accomplishment, but as we age, neither are we programmed to disintegrate into useless bags of protoplasm. Despite the many concerns raised by the coming centenarian surge, there are reasons to celebrate the extended impact these beautiful minds will make. Many of our oldest and brightest stars are far from being our dimmest. They're creating and contributing far deeper into their long lives than ever before.

Few epitomize this tirelessness quite like the indefatigable Dr. Jane Goodall.

At ninety, she's far from achieving centenarian status. But she's still working. The renowned British primatologist and conservationist has told her team she wants to learn something new every day. She engages with millions via Zoom and hosts a chart-topping podcast. "We call her Jane 3.0," a member of her inner circle says.

In 2021, Goodall won the prestigious Templeton Prize, which honors individuals whose life's work embodies a fusion of science and spirituality. Born in London in 1934, she traveled to Kenya in 1957 and met the famed anthropologist and paleontologist Louis Leakey. In 1960, at his invitation, she began her groundbreaking study of chimpanzees in what is now Tanzania. Her field research revolutionized the discipline of primatology, helping transform how scientists and the public perceive the emotional and social complexity of animals. She was the first to observe that chimpanzees—our closest evolutionary cousins—engage in activities previously believed to be exclusive to humans, such as creating tools, and she demonstrated that they have individual personalities.

She founded the Jane Goodall Institute in 1977 to sustain the study and protection of chimpanzees while also improving the welfare of scores of local communities. In 1991, she established Roots & Shoots, an environmental and humanitarian program whose hands-on projects have benefited communities, animals, and the environment in more than sixty-five countries.

Accustomed to traveling 300 days a year, she found herself confined to her childhood home in Bournemouth, England, when the 2020 coronavirus pandemic hit. That could have been reason enough to call it a career. Instead, she reinvented herself on social media, expanding her influence by many millions. "Virtual Jane," she calls herself.

In a wide-ranging interview for this book, she talked candidly about not just her desire but her visceral *need* to work—to have purpose, to give back, to contribute to the greater good.

"It seems I'm working harder than I worked in my entire life," says Goodall, whose grandmother lived to ninety-eight, her father to ninety-seven, and her mother to ninety-six. "I think I have more stamina now than I had when I was thirty. There's so much to do. I'm getting older, and that means there's less time. I'm caring for the environment, protecting endangered species, worrying about climate change and loss of biodiversity. I've been blessed with

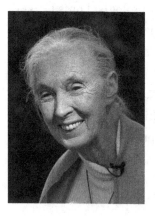

Celebrated primatologist Dr. Jane Goodall embodies what life can be in the tenth decade and beyond. (*Photo © Nick Stepowyj via Creative Commons*)

good genes, but I've just got to do more because there's less time to do it in. Even if I live to be 100, there'll be still massive problems to tackle. Things are so tough right now, and there are problems, which seem to be lacking solutions. I'm definitely going to keep on as long as I can. I have to. I can't stop." (More from Goodall in chapters 5 and 10.)

To help keep herself going, she's traded her nearly lifelong vegetarian lifestyle for a stricter vegan regime. And she takes brisk thirty-minute walks on the beach each day with her elderly sixteen-year-old whippet.

"I mean, I feel incredibly healthy," she says. "Aging hasn't worried me, and death itself holds no fear for me at all. At a big lecture, somebody asked me what my next adventure would be. I'd never been asked that before. Maybe ten years ago I would have said, 'Well, I want to go into the wild, unexplored jungles of some faraway country.' But now, no. So, I said, 'Well, dying.' And there was a kind of gasp that went around this huge auditorium. But when you die, there's either nothing, in which case I don't have to worry anymore, or there's something. And if there's something, which I happen to believe, then what an adventure it'll be to discover what that is."

For now, though, her thoughts are firmly among the living: specifically, keeping her fellow humans alive as long as possible and helping them thrive in a world she describes as "a very, very dark tunnel filled with obstacles."

"A lot of people just sit around and hope something will happen. But the key thing now is if we lose hope, that's the end."

.   .   .

How long can we live? How long *should* we live? These are fast becoming the great questions of life. And the answers, perhaps not surprisingly, are proving elusive.

Despite the uncertainty that awaits our swiftly aging society, most of us, unsurprisingly, want all the time we can get. Our lust for life comes through loud and clear in a 2022 survey conducted jointly by National Geographic and AARP, which asked more than 2,500 respondents this tantalizing question: *Assume for a moment that there was a pill that could extend your life by ten years. How likely would you be to take that pill?*

Three in four of those surveyed across all age groups said they'd happily swallow. But intriguingly, those aged eighty and up were the least likely to feel that way. Querying the octogenarians further, the researchers' suspicions were confirmed: Sure, extreme longevity is great, but only if accompanied by vitality, mobility, and independence. Some of the oldest of us, having begun to experience the loss of one or more of those, can't help but question the point of an extra decade. Others, flashing fierce determination and resilience, challenge the notion that it's a zero-sum proposition: 100 years, or vibrant health, but not both. Reality lies between those extremes, and for many of us, it'll probably look like a participant of the NatGeo/AARP study who's in her nineties and fast closing in on triple digits—a woman who still plays table tennis and sings in her church choir despite using a walker. "Good health," she says, "is being able to get up each day, and do the things that you plan to do, and not dread them."

That's a refreshing and appealing attitude. Unfortunately, popular culture hasn't always respected our oldest citizens. Jeanne Calment herself lived through nearly a quarter-century as a caricature, not unlike the ugly, witchlike old women unflatteringly depicted in a pair of Lewis Carroll classics published just a few years before her birth: *Alice's Adventures in Wonderland* and *Through the Looking Glass*.

Just a little more than a century ago, as World War I drew to a close, our life expectancy was merely half of what it is today. Tragically, sixty-one, my age today, remains the life expectancy at birth for people in Angola, the Democratic Republic of Congo, Mozambique, Togo, and much of sub-Saharan Africa. My gut, which is growing, says there's no way I'm potentially only half done, even as the grandson of a centenarian. But science won't rule it out. Jeanne Calment is proof of that.

So, how did we get here anyway?

CHAPTER TWO

HOW SCIENCE
LENGTHENS OUR LIVES

What I remember most about my uncle Andy was that he had the most lively and expressive brown eyes I've ever seen.

A World War II veteran and successful aviation engineer with an easy smile and Hollywood matinee idol good looks, Andrew P. Sansone left us far, far too soon. A congenital heart defect felled him at forty-seven, in the prime of his life, leaving behind a wife, four young children, and a heartbroken mother who nonetheless somehow marshaled the will to live very nearly to 104.

That woman was my maternal grandmother, Marie Mercurio Sansone. She was born to a Sicilian immigrant couple in 1899 in Brooklyn, New York, and died in 2003 after a life that touched three centuries—an impressively long run tinged with the sorrow of burying a child. Uncle Andy's premature passing was, and still is, a tragedy in our family. His sudden loss in 1972 was the second death I fully experienced. The first was my Grampa Joe, an affable, Sicilian-born grocer and house painter who succumbed to prostate cancer at sixty-seven, when I was just seven. I vividly recall my mother bolting from the dinner table, bawling, and running to my parents' bedroom after getting the dreaded call. That night, I cried myself to sleep.

Andy's death hit differently, if only because it caught us all so horribly off guard. I was eleven, with an adolescent's sensitivity, paranoia, and hypervigilance, and my centenarian-to-be grandmother, who was living with us at the time, was inconsolable. "Not my Andy! Not my Andy!" she wailed. Her grief, and my mother's, made me wonder if my own dad was next.

This cold fact will provide little comfort to my cousins, who grew up fatherless, but for centuries, forty-seven was a full life. In 1900, it was the average life expectancy at birth for Americans.

Cardiologists believe we're on the verge of virtually eliminating premature heart disease deaths. Some see us using the gift and power of science to identify people like my uncle Andy before they're even born and to make a few life-extending tweaks to their DNA in the womb, sparing nearly everyone the fate of sudden cardiac death.

It's already happening, and it's the latest example of how science lengthens our lives. In the last century alone, our life spans have doubled. Here's how it all went down—or up, in this case.

IN THE BEGINNING, OUR LIVES WERE FURTIVE, DESPERATE, AND shockingly brief.

Forget for a moment about centenarians. Thinking back eons through prehistory, they'd have been as mythical as unicorns. The average life expectancy of our earliest ancestors was capped at just ten years. In fact, anthropologists think our species survived enormous odds only because those who reached sexual maturity reproduced at twice our modern birth rate. Our staying power was in our numbers.

But we had something else going for us: our brains. They were smaller than they are now, yet proportionately much larger than those of the hyenas, giant crocodiles, and other toothy carnivores stalking us. We seemed to grasp the truth instinctively: Science—first expressed in our ability to make and control fire; later in our knack for fashioning crude tools from stone—was a lifesaver.

As the millennia ticked by, our early efforts to lengthen our life spans through science were neither inspired nor enlightened. We bled patients to cure their ailments. We treated people with mental disorders by drilling holes in their skulls. We gave our kids cough syrup laced with heroin. We fed our colds, starved our fevers, then argued over whether it should have been the other way around.

Yet through trial and error, blunders and breakthroughs, we prevailed. Evolution's genetic mutations favored our reasoning and resourcefulness, positioning us for long-term success. Today, despite the ravages of the coronavirus pandemic, average life expectancy at birth hovers at just under eighty years, and as we've seen, there's an unprecedented surge in the numbers of people living to well more than 100 just around the corner.

How did we go from ten to 100 and beyond? Fasten your seat belts (yes, those, too, have lengthened our days) for a ride back in time.

OUR FIRST STOP: 1764. ENGLAND WAS LAYING THE GROUNDWORK for its nearly two-century conquest of India; America's increasingly restive colonists were thumping their chests at the British crown; and an eight-year-old musical prodigy, Wolfgang Amadeus Mozart, was performing for King George III.

Newborns, on average, could expect to live thirty-four years, though some lived twice that or more.

In Cambridge, Massachusetts, Ebenezer Storer clung stubbornly to his faith, even as he walked through the valley of the shadow of death. But his stoic journal entry for March 11, 1764, still reads like a postcard from the edge of the world.

Earlier that day, the Congregational deacon had arranged for his children to be inoculated against smallpox, far and away the number one killer of his time. And his unease with this strange new practice—intentionally injecting them with a trace amount of the very virus that was ruthlessly sickening and killing millions—was palpable. You can feel his anguish in the prayer he scribbled by candlelight in a spidery hand:

> As it has pleased God in his sovereign providence to permit that contagious distemper the smallpox to spread in the town, I have this day caused my dear children with several others in my family to receive it by inoculation, humbly depending on Almighty God for success.
>
> O Almighty God, the author of our beings and the Father of our spirits, I humbly and earnestly look up to Thee on this day of distress & calamity.

Storer's deep unease was understandable. Early smallpox inoculations, while effective in many, put others into early graves. One pamphlet that circulated at the time denounced inoculation as "a delusion of the Devil."

Another demanded to know: "If Infection is communicated to another by means of Self-Infection, and this Contagion spreads itself among others, and any of these thus infected perish, at whose hands shall their Blood be required?"

But Storer's instinctive trust in medicine wasn't misplaced: His entire family recovered, and he himself lived to seventy-eight, an exceptional life span in the late eighteenth century.

As our new age of extreme longevity dawns, it's no accident that our life spans are extending deep into triple digits, with no hard limit in sight. And overcoming smallpox was one of the first vital hurdles.

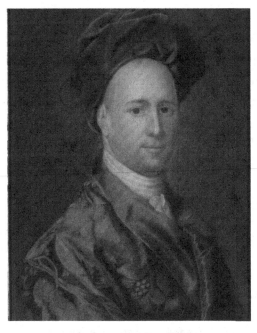

This John Singleton Copley painting depicts Ebenezer Storer, who bravely had his children inoculated against smallpox. (*John Singleton Copley via Creative Commons*)

By any measure, across every scientific discipline, smallpox was The Big One. In modern memory, it's killed as many as half a billion; 300 million since 1900. When the Pilgrims came ashore in 1620, they loaded their flintlock rifles with fresh gunpowder and lead musket balls and braced for spirited resistance from the native people, only to find their landing place a virtual ghost town: Three years earlier, the indigenous Wampanoag were laid waste by an outbreak that ravaged the tribe, and many historians think smallpox was the culprit. Pilgrim leader William Bradford, who would become the colony's first governor, recorded the desolation his scouts had discovered: "Skulls and bones were found in many places lying still above ground, where their houses and dwellings had been; a very sad spectacle to behold."

Smallpox was a clear and present danger throughout human history. Rashes and scars found on Egyptian mummies suggest it was a deadly scourge for at least 3,000 years, and very likely much longer than that. The earliest written description of a disease like smallpox appeared in China in the fourth century CE (Common Era). Early written descriptions also appeared in India in the seventh century CE and in Asia Minor in the tenth century CE. Some medical historians believe it wiped out the ancient Aztec and Inca civilizations.

It was a dreadful way to die. Infected people first experienced mild flu-like symptoms, but soon developed hundreds of fluid-oozing blisters all over their bodies. One in three perished. Those lucky enough to survive were left scarred or blinded for life.

Enter Edward Jenner, an English country doctor with a hunch that changed the world.

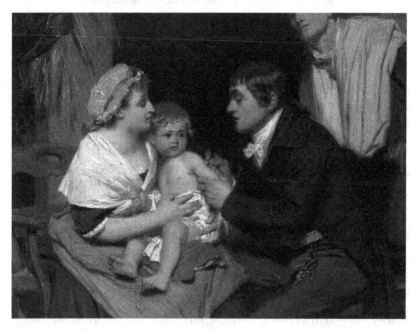

This painting by E. E. Hille shows Edward Jenner vaccinating a baby. (*E. E. Hille via Creative Commons*)

As a boy, he'd encountered milkmaids whose exposure to cowpox, a far less lethal livestock disease, appeared to give them a measure of protection against smallpox. In 1796, tweaking the technique that saved Storer and his family in 1764, Jenner vaccinated James Phipps, the eight-year-old son of his gardener, with a trace amount of cowpox. It was a stroke of genius—a scientific advance of epic proportions—although the ethics of his experimentation on a vulnerable child are still hotly debated today. Exposed later to smallpox, little James was immune. He'd grow up to marry, father children, and live out his days in a tidy brick cottage that Jenner leased to him for free, eventually dying at sixty-five.

NOT EVERYONE EMBRACED THE VACCINE'S VIRTUES. IN A BIZARRE 1721 example of backlash, someone tossed an explosive device into the home of the Reverend Cotton Mather, one of his era's most influential ministers and an active proponent of inoculation. It didn't explode, but a menacing message was attached: "Cotton Mather, you dog, damn you! I'll inoculate you with this; with a pox to you."

None other than founding father Benjamin Franklin was an avowed anti-vaxxer before he came to embrace inoculation after paying a terrible price: the death of a young son.

"I lost one of my sons, a fine boy of four years old, by the smallpox taken in the common way," Franklin wrote in his autobiography. "I long regretted bitterly and still regret that I had not given it to him by Inoculation; This I mention for the sake of parents, who omit that Operation on the Supposition that they should never forgive themselves if a child dies under it; my Example showing that the Regret may be the same either way, and that therefore the safer should be chosen."

The fight to contain smallpox, and the early struggles to understand how it spread, inspired poets and novelists, and their work occasionally bordered on ghoulish. In her 1744 novel, *The Adventures of David Simple*, writer Sarah Fielding—spinning a plot worthy of a Stephen King thriller—exploited a bit of eighteenth-century fake news: Smallpox could be contracted by fear, making timid women especially vulnerable to infection.

Buoyed by the undeniable efficacy of smallpox vaccinations, the British government tried in the late 1800s to make them compulsory. Protests and noisy blowback ensued, not unlike today's fringe resistance to vaccines and the dim view some contemporary skeptics take of governments they deem meddling and interventionist.

It would take another century and a half, but the last outbreak of smallpox in the United States was documented in 1949. In 1980, the World Health Organization declared the disease eradicated.

FAST-FORWARD EXACTLY A HUNDRED YEARS FROM 1764 TO 1864. Abraham Lincoln was reelected; the Geneva Conventions gave us wartime rules for treating our enemies; and China's bloody Taiping Rebellion wound down. By now, the average newborn could expect to live to forty-three.

Long live us all, but if we're going to lift a glass to twenty-first-century longevity, *"Vive la France"* will always be an appropriate toast.

Exactly a century after Ebenezer Storer had his children inoculated in fear and trembling, French chemist Louis Pasteur developed a technique to kill harmful bacteria in wine. Pasteur's motivation was untainted Merlot, but two decades later, a thirsty world pivoted to milk. Using the same technique, scientists began "pasteurizing" milk, dramatically decreasing disease and death from germs in raw dairy products. Millions were sickened and killed before pasteurization; today, such deaths are practically nonexistent.

In the mid-nineteenth century, though, the simple acts of eating and drinking could do us in.

Something food-borne and microscopically tinier than an assassin's bullet took out US president Zachary Taylor. On July 9, 1850, the nation's twelfth president died after eating food likely contaminated with salmonella bacteria at a Fourth of July picnic. For a very long time, enteric disease—illness contracted from tainted food or drink—was our Waterloo. During the Civil War, twice as many combatants died of food- or water-borne disease than of battle wounds. Typhoid, diarrhea, dysentery, and malaria were so rampant, they were collectively called "the third army"—even more lethal than the muskets, daggers, and cannons wielded by Union and Confederate forces who fought to the death in watery, bacteria-laden trenches where infected mosquitoes laid their eggs.

Among the casualties of this invisible menace was fifteen-year-old Joseph Beall Welsh. In 1862, the young Ohioan joined the Union Army. In a letter to his sister, he wrote: "You ought to see the Mississippi River. How would you like to drink that water where you could see 3 [dead] men floating down at one time?" Two years later, Welsh himself would die of typhoid fever, spread through contaminated food or water.

Chlorinating water to neutralize amoebas carrying dysentery and other parasitic illnesses was another life-extending advance. In 1908, Jersey City, New Jersey, became the first US metropolitan area to routinely disinfect community drinking water. The impact was instantaneous: The Centers for Disease Control and Prevention says cases of frequently fatal cholera and typhoid plunged dramatically. Combined with filtration, scientists found that chlorination reduced overall mortality by 13 percent. It was especially a lifesaver for children, cutting infant mortality by 46 percent and youth deaths by 50 percent.

We'd made impressive progress, but world wars and global pandemics slowed our march to 100.

In 1900, the average life expectancy for an American woman was 48.3 years; for a man, two years less. In 1918, as World War I ended and the Spanish influenza outbreak raged, that tumbled to 42.2 years for women and 36.6 years for men. Let that sink in for a second. If you're in your mid-thirties or early forties today, you may well have been done—deprived of life's biggest prizes: love and time itself.

ONWARD TO 1928. STALIN TURNED PEASANTS' LANDS INTO COLLECtive farms; Charles Kingsford Smith completed the first transpacific flight; and the Academy Awards made its glittery debut. By now, the average newborn could expect to live sixty-one years.

The discovery of penicillin was a huge leap forward: a veritable medical moon shot. And with it, our lives lengthened virtually overnight.

A splotch of the original mold that saved us is on display at the Smithsonian Institution. It's round, gray, flat, and fuzzy—exactly what Dr. Alexander Fleming, the grandfather of modern antibiotics (and his era's Neil Armstrong in our lunar landing metaphor), stumbled upon in his lab.

Penicillin's discovery was pure scientific serendipity. Returning from a two-week vacation, Fleming checked on the staphylococcus bacteria he'd been growing, and noticed a petri dish he'd absent-mindedly left out on a bench was contaminated by a mold that killed everything near it. Gwyn Macfarlane, a British hematologist, declared the find "a series of chance events of almost unbelievable improbability."

A God thing, Ebenezer Storer might have called it, had he lived in our time.

The first person to be given penicillin was Albert Alexander, a forty-three-year-old policeman in Oxford, England, whose body was riddled with infection after being injured in a Nazi bombing raid. Twenty-four hours after the first dose, his doctors noticed a startling improvement. But it was February 1941, World War II was raging, and the medical team's meager supply ran out before the cop could be cured. They even extracted the excess penicillin from their patient's urine and reinjected it into his veins, but he relapsed and died a month later.

Even so, the National Institutes of Health hails Fleming's epiphany as "the beginning of the antibiotics revolution," and it's credited with saving untold millions of lives worldwide. Before penicillin, infections like pneumonia, rheumatic fever, and syphilis often were death sentences. With the wonder drug, they became unpleasant setbacks.

"When I woke up just after dawn on September 28, 1928, I certainly didn't plan to revolutionize all medicine. . . . But I guess that was exactly what I did," the Scot later said. The Nobel Committee for Physiology or Medicine agreed: In 1945, it awarded Fleming and two associates the prize for that category.

The delay between Fleming's epic life-extending discovery and its widespread use is heartbreaking. His paper describing the

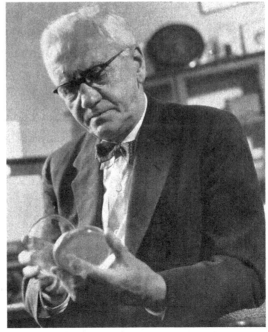

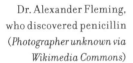

Dr. Alexander Fleming,
who discovered penicillin
(*Photographer unknown via
Wikimedia Commons*)

wonders of penicillin, first presented to the Medical Research Club at Middlesex Hospital early in 1929 and published the following year, languished in academic obscurity for years. It took a decade for penicillin to be purified for clinical use, and another before it was widely used as a shield against premature death. One can't help but wonder how many millions of lives might have been saved had there been better coordination and a greater sense of urgency.

Penicillin inspired other drugs to conquer diseases that once ruthlessly shortened our lives: streptomycin to treat tuberculosis; chloramphenicol for cholera and typhoid; tetracycline for pneumonia; erythromycin for diphtheria; cephalosporin for ear infections; vancomycin for colitis.

"Better living through chemistry," DuPont sloganeers crowed way back in 1935, and they weren't wrong. Thanks to science, we've blazed an unmistakable path into the realm of super-aging.

AND THEN WE FIND OURSELVES IN 1956. SOVIET TROOPS STORMED into Hungary; the first transatlantic telephone cable was completed; and in Liverpool, England, schoolboy John Lennon started a band as "a bit of a lark." Newborn life expectancy was now seventy-one: more than double what it was in Ebenezer Storer's day.

Vaccine skeptics are nothing new. For centuries, a hesitant and sometimes hostile public has tapped the brakes on big breakthroughs. Some questioned the wisdom of interfering with God's will; others objected to vaccine mandates as assaults on personal liberties.

Gradually, though, science's golden age prevailed. Collectively, we reached enlightenment on October 28, 1956, heralded by, of all things, a lip curl and a pelvic thrust.

As cameras rolled live at CBS Studios in New York, Elvis Presley was vaccinated for polio backstage at *The Ed Sullivan Show*. Since the 1940s, the disease had disabled 35,000 people a year, mostly children, in the United States alone. A 1921 polio infection robbed Franklin D. Roosevelt, then thirty-nine, of the use of his legs. Avenging that loss later as president, FDR launched a national foundation that would morph into the March of Dimes, marshaling loads of pocket change and political will to find a cure.

In a primetime message to vaccine-ambivalent teens, Presley implored: "I ask you to listen." Ella Fitzgerald, Sammy Davis Jr., and Louis Armstrong helped ensure the message reached youths of color. Polio even inspired the iconic song "A Spoonful of Sugar" in the 1964 Disney film *Mary Poppins*. Songwriter Robert Sherman penned the line, "A spoonful of sugar helps the medicine go down," after his son described being given the oral polio vaccine at school, where a nurse squirted the medicine on a sugar cube.

It worked: In 1979, polio was declared eradicated in the United States, meaning it was no longer spreading regularly. That doesn't mean it's gone: It remains endemic in Afghanistan and Pakistan; a polio infection recently was detected in the Netherlands; and even in the United States it occasionally resurfaces. In mid-2022, an unvaccinated adult from New York City who contracted polio and developed paralysis became the first US case in nearly a decade, and the polio virus was detected in wastewater in at least four counties in the New York metropolitan area. But it's been reduced by more than 99 percent, and most Americans are vaccinated against it.

Presley's message was aimed squarely at young people. Perhaps unsurprisingly, their elders had no one who had anywhere near his celebrity advocating for them. Through much of the previous century, the aged were as dismissed and devalued as they were in Jeanne Calment's heyday, when efforts to vaccinate seniors were halting at best. Worldwide, compliance with recommendations for vaccinating children has been generally high, at least in most high-income countries, with 90 percent of youngsters getting the shots they need—partly because so many schools require it. But older adults? Not so much. Many elderly were unprotected against polio in the 1950s and 1960s, partly because the focus was on shielding children from its crippling effects, but also because of seniors' own complacency and skepticism; public health challenges in getting them access to the shots; and society's entrenched indifference toward older people.

That mid-1900s zeitgeist around aging was captured perfectly by one of Elvis's contemporaries, actor, teen heartthrob, and cultural icon James Dean. "Live fast, die young, and leave a good-looking corpse," he famously quipped. Tragically, the universe complied; he was only twenty-four when he was killed in a car crash.

Globally, life expectancy before vaccinations and antibiotics averaged fifty years, but these scientific marvels extended our lives by more than a quarter of a century in Europe, North America, and other parts of the developed world. Provided, of course, you were lucky enough to be born in those places. (More on the inherent unfairness of extreme longevity in chapter 4.)

OUR LATEST STOP ON A RIDE THAT NEVER ENDS: 2021. WE BATTLED a resurgent coronavirus pandemic; some Americans refusing to accept the outcome of the 2020 presidential election staged an armed insurrection on the Capitol; and, at ninety, *Star Trek* actor William Shatner became the oldest human to blast off into space. US life expectancy at birth tumbled to 76.4 years, the CDC says. (The United Nations projects it will rebound to 79.25 years in 2024.)

If our unseen killers were printed as FBI most-wanted posters, we'd instantly see how far we've come. In 1900, the leading causes of death were pneumonia, tuberculosis, and diarrhea—all communicable diseases. Today, they're heart disease, cancer, stroke, and COVID-19.

It may seem strange to contemplate a world where people living to 105, 110, or even older will be commonplace in just a few decades. After all, in 2020, the coronavirus pandemic cut overall life span for Americans by a year and a half—the largest single-year decline since World War II. It was even more brutal among people of color, robbing Latino Americans of three years of life span and taking very nearly the same from Blacks. To be sure, killers other than COVID-19 played a role: Drug overdoses contributed, especially for whites, and rising homicides were a small but significant reason for the decline in life expectancy among Blacks.

But statistically, keeping in mind the great arc of human history, all of that is merely a blip on the screen. Experts say centenarians occur in a remarkably stable ratio of one in five thousand worldwide. With or without COVID-19, street violence, or the opioids scourge, they're coming en masse, riding one of the biggest population waves in modern history. It's just math: science's twin sister.

Already, there are more than 90,000 centenarians in the United States alone. Their ranks are swelling as members of the Silent Generation advance into their nineties, and they'll spike dramatically when the fittest and oldest of the baby boomers—now in their mid-seventies—follow over the next twenty-five years. By 2050, demographers say, we'll have eight times more centenarians than we do now. Centenarians are the fastest-growing age group globally.

Science, working in tandem with the body politic, has given us safer workplaces, smoking cessation programs, and seat belts. Buckling up, the National Highway Traffic Safety Administration says, has saved nearly 375,000 lives since 1975 in the United States. But biology and chemistry, specifically, have enhanced the resilience and sheer endurance of the human organism in ways our forefathers couldn't have imagined.

.   .   .

HAVING CONQUERED, OR AT LEAST TAMED, THE LEADING KILLERS
of the past, what are we doing about today's biggest obstacles on the
road to 100: cancer and cardiovascular disease? Heart attack and
stroke take an estimated 18 million lives a year, and cancers kill
another 10 million annually. They're the next Big Ones.

Dr. Richard Regnante—a Massachusetts cardiologist friend of
mine in his early eighties who's spent more than half a century
looking after his patients' heart health—is confident science will
come through. For Regnante, extreme longevity is personal: His own
father, a longtime assistant state attorney general who emigrated
from Italy, didn't stop working until he was ninety-five, and he lived
to 104. The son, too, remains youthful, sailing his twenty-nine-
foot Freedom yacht with surgical precision around Rhode Island's
Narragansett Bay. The wind tousles his salt-and-pepper hair as he
daydreams of a longer and brighter future—one he suspects may be
just over the horizon.

In a faint but unmistakable Boston accent, Regnante posits a
question that hundreds of researchers are scrambling to answer:
"What if we could map out the gene sequencing for coronary artery
disease, and tweak a person's DNA while they're still in the womb to
spare them a heart attack or stroke at midlife or later?"

Scientists at Yale University are making rapid headway in this
very direction. Racing to identify genetic mutations linked to cardiovascular diseases, they've already published data on five genes and
are studying twenty others. The Yale researchers have set themselves
a somewhat morbid goal: to figure out why some people with a family
history of undiagnosed heart problems die abruptly and prematurely
or end up having to move warily through life on a "watch and wait"
footing. Genetic sequencing, the scientists say, gives such people
an opportunity to learn if they have a mutation in their DNA that's
strongly associated with a potentially fatal heart condition. Patients
with that information, the theory goes, could benefit from early and

potentially lifesaving treatment. It's a line of scientific inquiry that's still in its infancy, but the Yale team is now sequencing the genes of 250 heart patients a year, slowly but steadily gaining knowledge it hopes will power new ways to screen and treat people at risk—and extend their lives.

CRISPR, a genome editing technology, could also soon be used to alter human DNA to provide protections against heart disease that would last a lifetime. In 2022, Verve Therapeutics launched a human trial of a CRISPR-based therapy designed to alter a New Zealander's genetic code to permanently lower that person's cholesterol levels. It's all flashing yellow, of course, as ethicists urge extreme caution, five years after now-disgraced and imprisoned Chinese scientist He Jiankui stunned the world by announcing he'd created the first gene-edited children—two girls later dubbed "CRISPR babies."

At least half a dozen active trials of human gene therapy are underway, and while the results so far are inconclusive, gene editing to lessen the likelihood of people dying of heart attack or stroke—the ultimate longevity Big One, and the force that took my uncle from his family in his prime—is shaping up as an increasingly promising treatment option.

Doug Olson of Pleasanton, California, is an early success story: In 2010, doctors used an experimental gene therapy that reprogrammed some of his blood cells to treat his leukemia and, more than a decade later, there's no sign of cancer. "This is a cure, and they don't use the word lightly," says Olson, who turned seventy-seven in 2024. Up to a few years ago, he was still running half-marathons.

Cancer patients used to be left to reckon not only with their tumors but with months of recovery from painful, invasive surgery. Now there's immunotherapy, using a new class of drugs to boost the immune system's natural ability to spot and kill cancer cells. In 2019, the US Food and Drug Administration approved the first immunotherapy drug for breast cancer, which kills 685,000 worldwide each year. And a revolutionary new treatment for stroke patients known as endovascular thrombectomy, or EVT, is giving surgeons unprecedented access to the cerebral artery to extract deadly or debilitating blood clots that form in the brain. Though still not widely available, experts believe the procedure has the potential to save millions of lives.

The next Big Thing: an emerging class of experimental drugs known as radiopharmaceuticals that deliver radiation directly to cancer cells. Doctors using them report improved survival in men with advanced prostate cancer. Experts believe that in the decades to come, they'll become an important tool for targeting tumors that are inoperable or hard to reach.

AND THE MEDICAL ADVANCES KEEP COMING. IN LATE 2021, THE World Health Organization endorsed the world's first vaccine for malaria, which kills more than 400,000 people a year in Africa alone. Every two minutes, malaria kills a child under age five. Until now, our best defenses were primitive: mosquito nets and insecticides. WHO Director-General Tedros Adhanom Ghebreyesus, a man not given to hyperbole, calls it "a gift to the world," and Julian Rayner, director of the Cambridge Institute for Medical Research, explains why: "It's an imperfect vaccine, but it will still stop hundreds of thousands of children from dying."

Nothing in recent memory can compare to science's astonishing response to COVID-19. The rapid development of multiple, highly effective vaccines was a medical miracle. Yet it was undermined by the perplexing refusal of many to be vaccinated. Science can extend our lives, but only if we believe it and heed it. If we don't, it's worse than gambling with our life savings—it's like leaving life itself on the table. That's something worth mulling over as we tumble ever deeper into a black hole of globalized pestilence, with the threat of another pandemic forever lurking just around the corner.

How long can we live? It's a vexing question; one that science is still trying to answer.

Provocative new research by a team of Russian scientists analyzing blood cell counts in elderly subjects suggests the outer limit, if there is one, could be as old as 150. Dr. Nir Barzilai of the Albert Einstein College of Medicine in New York, who discovered the first "longevity gene" in humans, thinks the ceiling is closer to 115 years, based on his extensive study of Ashkenazi Jews aged 95 to 109.

The very latest research tamps down expectations. "It is certainly possible that someone will eventually surpass Jeanne Calment's record, but the data suggest that they will surpass it only slightly, and the chance of observing any individual living past a higher milestone—such as 125 or 130 years—is so small as to be negligible," data scientist Brandon Milholland and geneticist Jan Vijg say in a new study published in the journal *Nature Aging*. Then they dangle this enticing scenario: "Past centuries have learned that in science no possibility can ever be excluded, and new insights and more advanced technologies may emerge to radically extend the maximum life span of our species above and beyond the current limit."

Underscoring the scientific disagreement around that question, two leading longevity experts have made a bet. Steven N. Austad, codirector of the Integrative Center for Aging Research at the University of Alabama at Birmingham, believes the first person who will live to 150 is probably alive right now. S. Jay Olshansky, a leading expert on public health and longevity, doubts anyone will ever live more than a decade longer than France's 122-year-old Calment. Each has put $300 into an investment fund and signed a contract stipulating that the money and any returns will be paid to the winner, or his descendants, in 2150. Based on the growth rate of the fund so far, the beneficiaries of whoever prevails could end up pocketing several hundred million dollars in winnings. Austad says he's more confident than ever he'll win this wager, based on continuing medical breakthroughs. Olshansky insists it's a sucker's bet, while acknowledging there's no age at which death is certain, leaving open the possibility that life span records will continually, if not dramatically, be broken.

WE'VE SEEN HOW ADEPT WE'VE BECOME IN ELIMINATING OR HEALING ourselves of life-threatening illnesses. Now a fringe school of thought is edging steadily closer to the scientific mainstream: What if we treated age itself as a chronic but curable disease? What if we could live to 200 and beyond?

David Sinclair, a Harvard Medical School geneticist, has been pressing governments to declare aging a disease, on par with diabetes or Alzheimer's. His rationale: Even if we found a cure for cancer tomorrow, life expectancy at birth would increase by only 2.3 years. Meanwhile, most of the billions spent on research are devoted to individual illnesses. Proponents of longevity medicine, focused on living not only longer but healthier lives, want to see more of those research dollars.

Sinclair likens the emerging field to the early days of flight.

"Old biological age is not reported as a cause of death, but it remains the main reason why older adults die worldwide," he says. "The problem is that we've always thought of aging as something natural and unavoidable as opposed to a disease, but actually, aging is a medical condition."

No matter that the US Food and Drug Administration so far refuses to recognize aging as a treatable disease. Sinclair's team at Harvard, and researchers at the Buck Institute for Research on Aging in Novato, California, are pioneering applications for epigenetics— essentially, accessing cells' control systems to figure out how to turn specific genes on and off. In a study published in the journal *Nature*, Sinclair and his team cured blindness in mice by genetically altering the rodents' eyes.

"And it's a permanent reset," Sinclair told a 2021 symposium.

"In fact, the mice die old but with very young eyes, with perfect eyesight," he said. "We're finding in the field that you can reprogram most tissues. I don't know of a tissue in an animal that cannot be reprogrammed and set back 50 percent, 75 percent in their age. Imagine in the future we have that ability to reset our bodies—not just once or twice, but perhaps dozens or hundreds of times."

Is all this the making of a longevity Utopia where we all live forever? Or an ominous step toward a decidedly dystopian future?

Medical ethicists warn of the latter, and even proponents of scientifically driven longevity have their doubts. Buck Institute president and CEO Eric Verdin notes darkly that, for the first time, the United States and other Western nations are selling more diapers for adults than for children.

A Google spin-off called Calico Labs is developing life extension technologies, hoping to pioneer and profit from a twenty-first-century Fountain of Youth. Another company, Unity Biotechnology—bankrolled in large part by Amazon billionaire Jeff Bezos and PayPal cofounder Peter Thiel—also is working on drugs to conquer the effects of aging. And tens of billions of dollars in venture capital are being poured into other startups, forming the vanguard of a rapidly expanding and potentially lucrative longevity sector.

Researchers in aging at the Harvard Stem Cell Institute—advancing earlier studies that showed that elderly mice injected with the blood of adolescent mice grew biologically younger—have identified a rejuvenating protein, GDF11 (growth differentiation factor 11), which also happens to be present in our own bloodstreams. They've since founded Elevian, a pharmaceutical company with a singular goal: investigating potential commercial therapies using GDF11 to slow, stop, or even reverse the effects of stroke and other calamitous conditions that hasten human aging.

Such antiaging ventures have their fans, but also their detractors.

"There are many possible harms: Dictators might live far too long, society might become too conservative and risk-averse, and pensions might have to be limited, to name a few," says John Davis, a professor of philosophy at California State University, Fullerton. Davis points to an even more troubling outcome: Because all new technologies are prohibitively expensive to begin with, extreme aging may become the exclusive provenance of the rich.

Others, including renowned bioethics scholar Walter Glannon, worry that a planet of centenarians will cause overpopulation on an unprecedented scale, draining resources desperately needed by younger generations.

The late sociologist and philosopher Bruno Latour, a member of the French Legion of Honor and a fellow of the American Academy of Arts and Sciences, took a dim view of efforts to significantly lengthen our lives. At what cost? he wondered. More isn't necessarily better.

And then, denouncing reckless "longevity entrepreneurs" who claim to sell immortality, he invoked the late German-American political scientist Eric Voegelin: Fundamentally, Latour said, "they're confusing Earth and heaven—and losing both in the end."

Overshadowing all of this is a far more daunting challenge: reversing or at least slowing the effects of climate change, our most existential threat. Success offers us all an immediate longevity pay-off. Failure, as the saying goes, is not an option. As the Earth warms, our future is at best a paradox—long in the short term; short in the long term.

In acting so late, and repeatedly faltering, we're ignoring an inconvenient truth: Even if we hit all our carbon dioxide goals, our ailing and compromised planet may not be able to oblige. Ebenezer

Storer's era was biblically awful, but climate change has the potential to make smallpox seem in comparison like the common cold.

A recent study at the University of New Brunswick, Canada, suggests people living next to water may live longer lives. That makes sense. Previous research has shown that deaths from cardiovascular and respiratory illness drop by as much as 12 percent among city dwellers fortunate enough to live close to parks and other green spaces; not water, specifically, but nature nonetheless.

People residing within 250 yards of a river, a lake, or an ocean are 17 percent less likely to die of several common causes of death, particularly stroke and respiratory illnesses, concludes Dan Crouse, the lead researcher on the waterfront study. His theory: Merely gazing at the water and hearing the soothing cadence of the waves lapping at the shoreline has a calming effect that eases life-wrecking stress.

But Crouse didn't address the obvious question: What's the point of investing in expensive waterfront property if rising sea levels mean those of us perched perilously near the coastline—like where my wife and I live in coastal Rhode Island—are going to drown?

Having overcome so much, positioning ourselves to join the giant sequoia, Galapagos tortoise, and bowhead whale in the pantheon of Earth's oldest organisms, are we really going to blow it by ignoring the groans of a planet in peril?

As if that's not enough, we're all looking down the barrel of another immediate and self-inflicted threat to life, limb, and longevity. Mass shootings and other gun violence—that uniquely American scourge—are becoming near-daily events. Unless and until we can find a way to limit ready access to military-style automatic rifles and high-capacity magazines, we're all in clear and present danger.

* * *

LIKE IT OR NOT, LIVING TO 100 AND BEYOND ISN'T MERELY WITHIN our grasp. Demographically and genetically speaking, it's a fate that awaits many of us.

Some of us will attain extreme ages we never asked for, let alone wanted. Others, desperate for more time, will leverage our life savings and jump the queue for every possible advantage.

We're in for a remarkable run, but some troubling thoughts necessarily take shape. Who's going to take care of us when we're all 100? Where will we come up with the cash to pay a century's worth of bills? How will our exceptionally longer lives play out for each of us?

We face some imminent and transcendent decisions here, and we must let history be our guide.

Think back for a moment to Alexander Fleming's accidental discovery of penicillin, and the two decades of inaction that tragically followed before the full force and fury of his microbiological weapon could be unleashed to keep us alive. For twenty years—an entire generation—millions of perfectly healable human beings needlessly coded on hospital gurneys, sheets pulled over their faces as grief-stricken families mourned losses that could have been prevented. Hindsight is 20/20, but in this instance, the future offers us a vision of what could be, and we'd best grasp hold of it. The likelihood that many of us will live to 100 is at hand. We can ignore extreme aging and let it ambush us, or we can heed the advice of the planet's most perceptive experts in the pages that follow and position ourselves—and future generations—to make the most of the time we're gaining.

Will we go out with a grin like Japan's Chitetsu Watanabe, who was the world's oldest man when he died at 112, outliving my equally affable uncle Andy by nearly two and a half times? His secret to longevity, he liked to say, was smiling, and his family was his joy: five children, twelve grandchildren, sixteen great-grandchildren, and a great-great-grandchild.

Or will we fade from view with a frown like so many of our eldest elders, vastly outliving our spouses, our children, and our friends?

As we careen toward a future few of us thought possible, a whip-sawing mix of bleakness and brightness, hope and despair, may be the best we can wish for. Most of us are destined to live long enough to at least double my uncle's forty-seven years, and then some. On the flip side, scientists warn, forty-seven years from now—in 2070—more than one in three people around the planet will be enduring "near-unlivable" temperatures as hot as those in the Sahara.

No matter how we'll eventually experience our 100s, Dr. Thomas Perls, America's foremost expert on centenarians, has a stark warning: We're aging on an unprecedented scale.

But let's forget the hype about a "silver tsunami"—that's negative imagery implying damage and destruction. I've come away brightened and inspired by every encounter I've ever had with a centenarian, and I prefer more positive phrasing to characterize what's coming. Think of it instead as an incoming tide—one that, if we get this right, causes all boats to rise.

Either way, you can be sure of this: The first waves already are lapping at our feet.

CHAPTER THREE

THE LUCK OF THE (DNA) DRAW

The old man's arteries surely begged for mercy. Or maybe not. Extreme longevity is funny that way. It can ignore clean living and seemingly reward bad behavior. People who break all the rules occasionally escape retribution.

We'll probably never know how or why my friend David Schultz's great-grandfather lived to just shy of 106, but David has two vivid memories of the man: Right up until his death, Robert L. Bowyer hauled the trash to the curb every day, and he liked to drizzle bacon grease instead of maple syrup on his pancakes.

Susanna Mushatt Jones, who lived to 116, upstaged him in both age and diet; she ate four strips of bacon daily with eggs and grits right up to her death in 2016 in Brooklyn, New York, and long had a sign in her kitchen that read: *"Bacon makes everything better."*

Their gloriously vibrant, long lives provoke vexing questions: How much does genetics contribute to longevity as opposed to things we can control such as diet, sun exposure, and exercise? Is living deep into our 100s a crapshoot, or are more methodical and measurable dynamics at play?

Admittedly, as a journalist, I have more questions than answers. So, I sat down with a respected, renowned scientist who's devoted most of his own life trying to understand what makes the very oldest of us tick. In the course of our many conversations, we discovered to our mutual delight that we share a lifelong obsession with Jeanne Calment.

FROM THE NINTH FLOOR OF AN IMPOSING BRICK BUILDING ON THE fringes of the Boston University campus, one of the world's most respected authorities on centenarians and supercentenarians is working to decode the secrets of their longevity.

Dr. Thomas Perls runs the New England Centenarian Study, the largest of its kind in the world. He and his team have studied 2,500 centenarians—including about 200 who have reached or exceeded the supercentenarian age of 110 or older, and another 600 "semi-supercentenarians" who have made it at least to 105. They've also studied 800 centenarian offspring, plus some spouses who don't have extreme longevity running in their families and serve as a sort of control group. So far, they've identified 281 specific genetic markers that are predictive of an epic life span.

Lean and boyish for a new grandfather, Perls—an international leader in the field of gerontology, which really came into its own just a little more than a century ago—smiles easily, wears aviator sunglasses, and makes liberal use of the smiley emoji in his emails. Ever the scientist, though, he speaks haltingly and chooses his words carefully.

With the ranks of US centenarians already expanding rapidly and profoundly, Perls's study until recently turned away applicants unless they were at least 103. "These are not people who are used to being told they're too young for anything," he says. "The number of centenarians is definitely getting much higher, and it's going to get much, much higher as the baby boomers start heading there."

Now, with a staff of twenty-five; partnerships with UCLA, Georgia State University, and the Albert Einstein College of Medicine in New York; and a new $25 million grant from the National Institutes of Health to study Alzheimer's in centenarians, Perls can enroll anyone 100-plus. But it's that subset of people who've made it to 105 and beyond that intrigues him most. They hold the keys to exceptional longevity that may unlock it for the rest of us.

"We've really concentrated lately on trying to recruit and enroll as many of these most extreme individuals because we regard them as our crème de la crème," Perls says. "The centenarians who live to 100 or 101 are a pretty mixed group. All of them greatly delay the onset of disability, but they're what we call *different phenotypes*. They're different kettles of fish. And yet when you start looking at people 105 and older, they begin to look really alike. We think the pathways, or mechanisms, of what are getting people to 100 can be pretty different. That's especially the case for the ones who go to 110 and older.

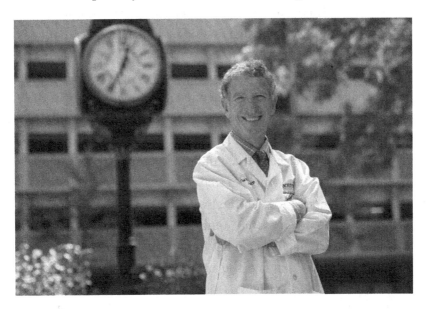

Dr. Thomas T. Perls, founder of the New England Centenarian Study (*Cydney Scott / Boston University Photography*)

And if they're phenotypically getting much more alike, then they're probably genetically and biologically much more alike as well, which means you need fewer of them to make these discoveries. Instead of many thousands of people getting to 100, just a few thousand people, say, getting to 105 and older may be what we need to make some of these discoveries."

Over more than three decades devoted to studying these extraordinary humans, all of whom are immeasurably older than himself, Perls has decoded some of their secrets. And it mostly comes down to DNA.

So far, he's found, each of those 281 genetic markers associated with a triple-digit life span has three variations. They involve at least 130 genes, many of which have been shown to play roles in Alzheimer's, diabetes, heart disease, high blood pressure, and various forms of cancer. Hitting enough of those to make it to 100 is like winning all five lottery numbers plus the Powerball, and that's especially true of those like Calment who catapult their way to 110 or beyond—something just one in 5 million of us manages to pull off.

Other researchers have been focusing on specific "longevity genes" that appear to protect centenarians against key age-related diseases. Dr. Nir Barzilai, who oversees the Longevity Genes Project at the Albert Einstein College of Medicine in New York City, sees the greatest promise in a gene that tamps down the body's production of human growth hormone. Barzilai notes that, in general, smaller animals live longer and healthier lives than larger ones: More compact dog breeds, for instance, tend to outlive larger breeds. One in two centenarians, his team has found, has a gene in the growth hormone pathways that taps the brakes on height and weight. In a new study, they used antibodies to block growth hormone in mice, and the rodents who were given that therapy lived 15 percent longer. Barzilai, who cofounded a biotech company that's been developing mitochondria-based therapeutics to treat diseases associated with aging, tells the Milken Institute Center for the Future of Aging that he feels a sense of urgency: "We should start targeting aging and start developing the drugs now. . . . We have to move fast."

But there are other factors that scientists are still working to unravel. One of these is that exceptional longevity seems to run in families. Male siblings of centenarians are seventeen times more likely to live to 100, and female siblings eight times more likely, according to a Boston Medical Center / Boston University Medical School study that looked at centenarians' brothers and sisters to see how they fared.

When you encounter a centenarian—really, any human being of any age—you're looking at the outward expression of an internal and exquisitely complex genetic profile. What Perls and his team have found is that the older a person is, the more accurate genetic markers become in predicting extreme aging. Think of exceptional longevity as a puzzle that's slowly taking shape on your family room coffee table. As we grow older, the genetic piece gets bigger.

And it gets more interesting.

For instance, with a few rare exceptions, centenarians are just as genetically predisposed as the rest of us to develop the kinds of diseases we've come to associate with older folks—heart disease, stroke, cancer, and Alzheimer's. That's pointing researchers toward genetic variants that are linked to longevity. Just as some people have more HDL, or "good" cholesterol, than LDL, or "bad" cholesterol, and the ratios of those two things point toward a long life or an untimely death, the idea is that centenarians have a genetic makeup that gives them a survival advantage, one where beneficial, protective variants offset those that would put most of us on our deathbeds.

Groups of people with common DNA profiles share what are called genetic signatures. Nine in ten of the centenarians in the New England study have one of more than two dozen genetic signatures.

Some of those exceptionally old individuals include people who have managed to avoid heart disease altogether. Others ward off Alzheimer's until the last five or ten years of their lives, if it ever touches them at all. They face disease like the rest of us, but not only don't they die, they somehow manage to stave it off and function independently for decades.

This is what Perls means when he says: "The older you get, the healthier you've been."

Genes, of course, don't account for everything. Centenarians figure into that age-old predestination versus personal choice calculus that's bedeviled us since the dawn of time. What's more determinative of a 100-year life span—who we are at birth, or what we make of ourselves?

We may be genetically predisposed to live to 100 or older, but there's a growing body of evidence to suggest that our individual choices around diet, exercise, and sun exposure are part of the equation.

The key, longevity experts say, is not to expect too much from either diet or exercise, since it's the right combination of both that gives us an advantage. A new study published in the *British Journal of Sports Medicine* cautions against eating health foods like kale without also spending a little time—even just ten minutes—exercising vigorously each week. Likewise, the researchers found, embracing a gym-rat lifestyle won't mean much if we're eating fatty foods. "Adhering to both quality diet and sufficient physical activity is important" in reducing our risk of dying from cancer or cardiovascular disease, the British team concludes.

Perls has developed an online tool designed to take all of this into account and help us determine our chances of hitting triple digits. His Living to 100 Life Expectancy Calculator (you can try it yourself at his website, Livingto100.com) is designed to capture what he's learned from decades of studying centenarians and other life span research, and help individuals estimate their longevity potential. Among the questions it asks: What's stressing you out lately? Do you feel like you're getting enough sleep? How much caffeine, alcohol, and tobacco do you consume? How many days a week do you exercise? And a slew of medical history questions; notably this one: Do you have at least one relative who lived to 100?

I dutifully ran my own bona fides through the calculator, and it spit out a result that at once neither surprised me, as the grandson of a centenarian, nor was one I was exactly expecting: "Your calculated life expectancy is 102 years." To be honest, it was the fine print on the screen that really threw me: "You're going to live for 40 more years! Do you have enough money saved to live that long?" Yikes! (Much more on the financial implications of living to 100 in chapter 9.)

LIKE ALL OF US, I REFLECT A MYSTERIOUS MIX OF LIFESTYLE choices and genetics, and I'm still trying to grasp how those two dynamics can both compete with and complement each other. Scientists, too, are puzzling over precisely how these dynamics interplay, but they believe about 25 percent of the reason one person lives to 100 and another lives to, say, eighty is driven by genetic factors.

Clearly, whatever DNA I've inherited from my 103-year-old grandmother puts me at an advantage in terms of longevity. So does the DNA I've been handed down from my mother, who's ninety-two and still living independently in the suburban Boston house I grew up in. But the other branches of my family tree are truncated. My father died at sixty-seven, and one of my brothers at fifty-nine. I've already mentioned my uncle Andy, whom we lost at forty-seven. One of my grandfathers passed away at sixty-seven; the other at seventy-five. That's a pretty mixed bag, but it turns out it aligns well with the experiences of most American families: Women in general tend to outlive men, and there are far more female than male centenarians. Men in their sixties, like me, have a 3.4 percent likelihood of living to 100; women, a 6.5 percent chance.

If I *do* make it to 100, though, what will get most of the credit—my DNA or my lifestyle? The jury's out on that. Here's what I mean. You can substitute yourself for me in these scenarios, adjusting for your own dietary, exercise, and other health choices.

For starters, I'm an endurance athlete who's run a dozen and a half marathons and more half-marathons, 10Ks, and 5Ks than I can count. But it wasn't always like this. Between my youth, when I ran track and cross-country in high school and later as a mediocre walk-on at Boston University, and today, I spent fifteen years smoking a pack a day; sometimes two; and carried twenty pounds more than I do now. That decidedly unhealthy lifestyle crept in as I was working sixty-plus hours a week as a foreign correspondent, and my heaviest smoking and drinking coincided with the decade I spent hopping on planes to cover the combustible Balkans and the rest of eastern Europe—a richly cultured yet undeniably self-destructive part of the world where practically everyone seems to be bogarting a cigarette with one hand while knocking back a snifter of plum brandy with the other.

Fortunately for all of us, the human body—even when abused—has an extraordinary capacity to repair itself.

In my mid-forties, horrified at what I'd done to myself and mindful of my own father's early exit at sixty-seven, I took up running once more. By the time we returned to the United States, I was the proverbial lean, mean, running machine. I joined the storied Greater Boston Track Club, the same team for which my lifelong idol, the great marathoner and former American record-holder Bill Rodgers, once competed.

But not long after I turned fifty, something imperceptible but undeniable shifted, and within months, the wheels came off. Coach Tom Derderian, who sugarcoats nothing, articulated my experience perfectly, if brutally. "Look, Bill," he told me trackside as I leaned over, panting and trying mightily not to throw up after struggling in vain to keep up with athletes half my age, "you're gonna get older, and you're gonna get slower, and eventually, you're gonna die."

Fast-forward a decade, and those words (minus the death piece—gee, thanks, Coach, for the inspiring speech) have turned out to be painfully prophetic. In my forties, I ran daily, logging up to sixty miles weekly. Nowadays, in a concession to age and the need to recover between efforts, I run every other day, and rarely put in more than twenty miles a week. Make no mistake: I'm deliriously happy to still be able to lace up my running shoes and engage in the delicious, endorphin-inducing ballet of human movement. Never mind that I, once a hare, skipped the tortoise stage and went straight to a snail's pace. "Don't slip in my slime trail," I warn fellow runners. They chuckle, but I mean it.

Rocker Bruce Springsteen knows how I feel. Onstage during his first major tour in six years, the Boss told fans in Tampa, Florida: "At fifteen, it's all tomorrows. And at seventy-three, it's a whole lot of yesterdays. That's why you've got to make the most of right now."

Age can make itself felt much earlier. Just ask Kieran Culkin, the star of HBO's *Succession*, who tells *Esquire* magazine about turning forty: "Everything changed. Get a little paper cut on my finger; nine days later, why do I still have a paper cut? It's just fucking slow now."

And yet decrepitude doesn't happen to everyone. Mike Fremont, a 102-year-old vegan runner from Vero Beach, Florida, does pull-ups daily and runs five miles a few times a week; basically the same mileage I'm doing, and I'm four decades his junior. "These, believe it or not, are the best years of my life," he tells fitness author and podcaster Rich Roll. The retired civil engineer and climate activist set the American record in the ninety-five to ninety-nine age category for the mile when he was "only" ninety-six. And he's not alone. At 105, Louisiana track athlete Julia "Hurricane" Hawkins set a new world record in the age 105-and-up category for the 100-meter dash, clocking 1 minute, 2 seconds.

In all of this, two questions haunt me: Will exercise provide absolution for my earlier transgressions? And how much, if at all, will the way I'm wired genetically take up the slack?

Matters of diet and nutrition are even more murky. Despite her own vitality and longevity as the daughter of a centenarian, my mother's cholesterol levels have always been high—elevated enough that, for years, she's taken medication to lower them. My own levels, low for a blissfully long time, soared into the mid-200s, although the ratios between good and bad cholesterol have always been favorable. Recently, thanks to exercise and the virtues of a quasi-pescatarian diet heavy on fish and light on red meat, my total cholesterol is back under 200. And even though I no longer train for or competitively run marathons, my resting pulse hovers around fifty beats per minute (72 bpm traditionally is the average, though doctors say the healthy range can span 60 to 100 bpm, depending on age and other factors). Likewise, my mother, who no longer exercises, is still enjoying the accumulated benefits of a lifetime of exercise classes at the local gym and enough miles walking around her neighborhood or on the treadmill in her basement to rival all of my marathons.

So what? Does it matter? Fundamentally, what's more important: The fitness we work so hard to achieve and maintain, or the way we're wired genetically? Can our best efforts overcome our worst genetic destinies? Is extreme longevity a zero-sum game, a sliding scale, or something in between? When I devour a greasy bacon cheeseburger with fries, can I play the "grandma card"?

SCIENTISTS ARE STILL FIGURING IT OUT, BUT AFTER DECADES OF extensive research into the very oldest of us, Perls has determined that centenarians tend to fall into one of three categories: survivors, delayers, and escapers.

Forty percent of all centenarians, he says, live for more than twenty years with age-related diseases—mainly heart disease and cancer—usually associated with significant mortality. They're the survivors. Another 45 percent deal with such diseases after age eighty. They're the delayers. Then there's the 15 percent who have none of these diseases by the time they turn 100. They're the escapers. It's a relative term, of course: When it comes to death, we can run but we can't hide, and nobody gets out of this alive.

But if we can't live forever, what's the outer limit for an individual human being's existence? As we explored in the previous chapter, provocative new research suggests it could be as high as 150. Prominent aging experts still can't agree on whether there's a hard ceiling. But scholarly studies suggesting there isn't—including one in Italy that found that once we hit 105, the odds of death stop increasing—make a convincing case for what gerontologists call a "mortality plateau." Translation: Live long enough, and all bets are off.

Perls thinks so, too, though he believes there's no way we'll ever live to 150: "We fantasize about winning the Mega Millions lottery. We fantasize about living to 150 or 200. But that's what it is. It's fantasy. There's not much scientific basis to it."

In one of our conversations, he told me: "If you have a healthy centenarian who's cognitively intact with no signs of Alzheimer's, to me, they're practically immortal."

In an interview in his cramped Boston University office festooned with framed degrees and awards, he said, "Genetic wiring–wise, we're all very, very similar."

Recapping more than three decades of inquiry into the complexities of the centenarian genome, Perls notes that his own work, and that of others, shows that practically all of us not only share the same genes but the exact same variations. That's not to say, of course, that

we're carbon copies of one another: A small proportion of our genes
include variations that differentiate us—not merely in the way we
look and act, but in how we interact with our environments and, most
critically, in how we age. It's nothing special—Perls characterizes it
as "an average set of wiring"—but as humanity moves into the 2020s,
he says, it's good enough to get us to ninety, or pretty close.

Those of us who make it to ninety can mostly thank our behaviors.
In the 1980s and early 1990s, scientists in Scandinavia demonstrated that 70 to 75 percent of living that long was firmly rooted
in a healthy lifestyle. In the United States, a landmark study of the
Seventh-day Adventist religious denomination produced similar
results. Members don't smoke; they don't drink alcohol; they eat
nutritious meals; they exercise regularly; and they take seriously the
biblical admonition of a weekly day of rest, which helps them manage
stress. Their average life expectancy? Nearly a decade longer than
the average American: eighty-six for men; eighty-nine for women.
And that extra life span cuts across race, ethnicity, geography, and
socioeconomic status. A 2015 Pew Research Center study found
Seventh-day Adventists among America's most racially and ethnically diverse religious groups.

"Their approach ups the ante a lot," Perls says. "They're basically
saying people can live thirty years beyond the age of sixty, on average,
which is a huge chunk of time." It is intriguing that only one of the
world's so-called blue zones, where people supposedly live longer, is
in the United States, specifically Loma Linda, California, a base for
Seventh-day Adventists. (More on what's really happening, and not,
in blue zones in chapter 10.)

Invariably, when matters of diet come up, we can't help but question whether our sacrifices and self-denial are worth it. Writer Tom
Ellison captures that tension perfectly in a hilarious piece of satire
for *McSweeney's Internet Tendency* titled: "I've Optimized My Health
to Make My Life as Long and Unpleasant as Possible."

"I have not eaten cake since my sixth birthday. My lifestyle factors predict I will live at least 120 optimal, cake-free years," he grumbles.

That's the behavioral piece; the stuff we can control. It certainly enhances our chances of getting to ninety. But what happens after that point becomes increasingly dependent on genetics.

Not entirely, though. If you're fortunate enough to live into your late nineties and hit 100, and you have a brother or a sister, that sibling also has an increased chance of attaining an extreme age. Researchers long ago noticed and zeroed in on this familial component. Familial, however, isn't the same as genetic. Perls explains: "Family members have health-related and behavioral traits in common. For example, smoking runs in families. So do socioeconomic status, years of education, access to better health care. Those things can run in a family, too." Centenarians' offspring also carry genetic advantages. Children of people 100 or older, a Spanish study found, have a unique genetic profile that may help explain why they're comparatively less frail than the children of non-centenarians.

Scientists have discovered that aging more slowly—something that boils down to avoiding diseases associated with growing old—is extremely complex when it comes to the precise biochemical pathways that are involved. Remember those 281 genetic markers Perls and his team have identified? He now suspects as many as 500 different protective genetic variants may be playing subtle or more pronounced roles in shielding centenarians from the worst the world can throw at them, effectively slowing their aging by decreasing their risk for disease.

"That's one of the really exciting facets of our work," Perls says. "If you can find things that are protective, and then understand the underlying biological pathways that are leading to that protection—if you can develop drugs that do the same things as these genes—you may be making a dent in things like slower aging and decreasing the risk for certain aging-related diseases."

Most such drugs are years, if not decades, from being developed, approved by regulators, and made widely available. Meanwhile, what and how much we eat and how we treat our bodies are key factors in determining our individual chances of living to 100 or beyond—and getting there in relatively good health.

Perls and his team have found that diet and exercise account for 75 percent of what gets most of us to ninety, but for those who live substantially longer, the ratio flips. Only one in 5 million people live to 110, achieving supercentenarian status, and for those rare humans, it's 75 percent genetics, not clean living and a clear conscience.

"It really is a matter of getting the right combination. And that's very, very rare. Much less rare if it runs in your family because the genetics runs in the family," he says.

I mentioned earlier, to my everlasting shame, that I'm an ex-smoker. Will the changes I've made since quitting—regular vigorous exercise and a mostly clean diet—possibly offset my incredible stupidity and give the centenarian genes I presumably carry a decent shot at saving me from myself? Obviously, there are no guarantees, but imagine my relief when Perls tells me: Yes. Even some people with the genes to reach 100 who've compromised that built-in longevity by engaging in horribly destructive behaviors such as smoking, he says, essentially can salvage their birthright by quitting in their forties and fifties. Make no mistake: It's unfathomably better to never, ever light up; but if you're like me and ignored science, society, and your mother, there's still hope—provided you reverse course now, before it's too late.

Perls, incidentally, isn't optimistic that we'll make many more huge strides in improving the health of our heart and lungs. The big declines we've seen over the past half a century with decreased smoking, he believes, leave us little room for substantial reductions in heart disease. But cancer? That's another story, and it's a critical piece of the super-aging puzzle.

. . .

JUST THE TERM CAN RATTLE US. THE *C-WORD*, WE CALL IT, UNWILLING to fully articulate the human body's alarming ability to turn on itself, sometimes fatally, without warning.

But cancer, a leading cause of death, is also a part of life. More than 18 million of us worldwide were living with it in 2020, according to the London-based World Cancer Research Fund—most of those cases involving breast, lung, and colorectal cancer.

Fortunately, we're all benefiting from liquid biopsy, a newer technology that examines DNA fragments produced by cancer cells and released into the bloodstream. Those fragments are distinctive compared to what normal, healthy cells produce, and zeroing in on them is helping doctors detect cancer much, much sooner than previously possible, simply by drawing a blood sample. The consequences to life and longevity are enormous: A diagnosis of pancreatic cancer, for instance, frequently amounts to a death sentence, but until recently, that was mostly because it was detected so late. Liquid biopsy—essentially analyzing the blood for cancer's calling cards—can give doctors the jump very early on, greatly increasing a patient's chances of survival.

And the personalized treatments that have sprung from that work have become so commonplace and effective, primary care physicians increasingly are taking over cancer surveillance from oncologists. In many cases, cancer specialists don't need to re-involve themselves unless a patient's unique, mapped-out tumor marker reemerges or evolves. "For cancers often detected at a late stage, such as lung, pancreatic, and ovarian, [cancer biomarkers] could detect a typically terminal malignancy at an earlier, more treatable, even curable stage," says Nithya Krishnamurthy, the lead researcher on a study published in the *Journal of Clinical Medicine*.

Not that those of us destined to become centenarians necessarily need the help. Most people who get to 100 already have a significant resistance to cancer. But breakthroughs like liquid biopsy will help prospective centenarians overcome an encounter with cancer earlier in life and go on to fulfill their life span potential. So, too, will immunotherapy, which targets tumors by getting our cancer-killing T cells—a type of white blood cell that is part of the immune system—to work a little harder and more effectively, and new vaccines like one for human papillomavirus that's led to a staggering 65 percent drop from 2012 through 2019 in the incidence of cervical cancer among women in their early twenties—the first group to benefit from the HPV vaccine.

Such breakthroughs figure prominently in those startling projections by the Stanford Center on Longevity: that living to 100, a once-unattainable milestone, will become the norm for newborns by 2050.

Peering into the future, the Stanford researchers wax positively Utopian.

"Today's five-year-olds will benefit from an astonishing array of medical advances and emerging technologies that will make their experience of aging far different from that of today's older adults," they project. "As they age, these future centenarians might deploy technology functioning as 'smart skin' to monitor heart, brain, and muscle function for abnormal activity or disease. These bio-integrated electronic devices, thinner than a human hair and as supple as skin, could supplant today's wearable technologies (smart watches, Fitbits, and the like) and be capable of preventing an epilepsy attack, resetting an irregular heartbeat, or sending biometric data to be analyzed by a doctor for early intervention. Heart attacks and strokes could be diagnosed remotely in their earliest moments, possibly reducing severe organ damage and death. In the future, older adults will be able to remain mobile longer than they can now, with the help of thin, wearable exoskeletons that let them walk and run with enhanced strength, much as e-bike riders power uphill without huffing and puffing."

Already, the march to 100 is particularly evident in Hong Kong, which has the world's second-highest average life expectancy—85.96 years in 2024—trailing only tiny Monaco at 87.14. Against all odds, life expectancy there has risen since the coronavirus pandemic erupted, albeit incrementally. Hong Kong's life tables indicate that one in five women, and one in ten men, are positioned to reach 100. Not coincidentally, smoking is rare there, thanks to blatant advertising about its dangers, very high taxes on tobacco, and strict rules that forbid it in public places, even outdoors.

Comparing Hong Kong to the United States, Perls can't help but sigh. On one prominent global ranking of life expectancy powered by the World Bank and the World Health Organization, the United States ranks forty-sixth; on another, fifty-sixth. So much for American exceptionalism.

"You know, one of the reasons we rank so poorly in average life expectancy in the United States is because there's such a large portion of our population that takes such bad care of themselves. It just drags the average down," he laments. "Sixty percent of our population is overweight. We have too many people still smoking. We have too many people eating horrible things."

In recent years, some of those poor health trends have emerged even in Japan, which traditionally has produced strong numbers of supercentenarians. Gerontologists point to the Westernization of Japan, particularly among men. They've taken on Western diets; there's a lot more smoking; rates of high blood pressure are prevalent; and work-life balance has eroded as stress levels soar. Japanese men now have roughly the same likelihood as their American counterparts of living to 100. Japanese women fare better, with one in seven becoming centenarians.

All this stokes an intriguing, if somewhat provocative, theory in Perls's mind: "I think that when the dust settles, we're going to find that Asians somehow have a bit more genetic predisposition of getting to 100."

Hear him out: "You know, they tend to be short and thin, and there may be some hormonal and genetic things associated with that that are quite conducive to getting to a much older age. I don't think it's ever going to be simple. But, for example, we know that growth hormone is associated with earlier mortality. Things like heart disease and stroke and cancer and diabetes are associated with elevated growth hormone levels. Well, if you're shorter, you may well have lower growth hormone levels over the course of your lifetime, and certainly lower levels when you're older. And that may be conducive to getting to older age. That's a very simplistic possibility, and there's going to be many other things."

To get to the bottom of that, the New England Centenarian Study increasingly has been looking at a population of centenarians as racially and ethnically diverse as possible. Associates at Georgia State University have a subcontract in one of Perls's studies to recruit and enroll Blacks. Other partners at UCLA are subcontracted to focus their work on Latinos. And at Mount Sinai Hospital in New York, an associate is recruiting and enrolling Cantonese- and Mandarin-speaking centenarians and their siblings. By discovering genetic variants and biological pathways that cross ethnic and cultural lines, Perls says, his team can better grasp what's most important to all humans for living in health as long as possible, and also be alert for any special predispositions one race or ethnicity may have over another in terms of extreme aging. Ultimately, he says, what's learned is likely to lead to more precision medicine that will keep us alive not only longer, but in better shape.

Each centenarian has blood drawn and a comprehensive genetic profile drawn up. Medical history and dietary habits are carefully recorded. They also undergo a thorough cognitive assessment to detect the presence or onset of dementia or Alzheimer's, and MRI neuroimaging scans to get a snapshot of their brain, which is examined to see if their gray matter looks normal and healthy or is beginning to show telltale markers of Alzheimer's or other neuro-degenerative diseases. Spouses and siblings, if still alive, get the same. At regular intervals, more blood is drawn. If you're beginning to get the idea that gerontologists are medicine's vampires, you're not wrong. But there's a reason for that: Our blood is, in many respects, a blueprint of who we are.

Perls's team squeezes a lot out of a small sample of a centenarian's blood. They do what's known as genomics, analyzing the person's complete set of DNA as well as sequencing all of the protein-coding regions of his or her genome. They do transcriptomics, which involve gene expression studies—basically, looking at what turns on a specific gene to get it to make RNA molecules, something present in all living cells. They do metabolomics, zeroing in on a couple thousand different metabolites, substances made or used when the body breaks down food, drugs or chemicals, or its own tissue. They do proteomics, analyzing about 7,000 different proteins. And they do methylomics, examining the presence or absence of things called methyl groups that attach to our DNA and turn it on or turn it off. It's a different way of looking at gene expression. UCLA researcher Steve Horvath famously used the presence of those methyl groups to create "biological clocks"—ways of measuring a person's age not by years but with a biological assessment of just how much a person has aged.

And, more recently, the researchers are looking closely at, of all things, centenarians' poop.

Ever mindful of the key role that our genes play in getting us to extreme old age, the Boston researchers regularly collect stool samples from centenarians. Then they analyze the microbiome within—that mishmash of bacteria, fungi, viruses, and their genes, all of which naturally live both on our bodies and inside us—for specific bacterial populations that may be conducive to super-aging. Scientists say the microbiome in our gut produces substances that cross into our bloodstream and can dramatically influence whether we develop Alzheimer's and other aging-related diseases; in fact, new research in China suggests the microbiome may function as an antioxidant system in centenarians. For these reasons, Perls tells me, "We've pretty much gone gangbusters in terms of getting fecal samples on almost all of our subjects."

Finally, centenarians in his study continue to be examined even after they've passed away, for only then do some of them give up their greatest secrets.

When a centenarian dies, a specialist is dispatched to the funeral home to remove the brain—something all subjects agreed to when they entered the study—and sends it on ice to the neuropathology lab at UCLA. Once there, it's immediately processed: Half of the brain is flash-frozen using liquid nitrogen (not unlike the frozen berries, chicken breasts, fish fillets, and dinner rolls we buy at the supermarket), and the other half is placed in formaldehyde.

"With the frozen part, we can take chunks from different areas of the brain and send that to our colleagues, like at Beth Israel Deaconess [Medical Center] here in Boston, where they're looking at the expression of genes in very specific areas of the brain," Perls says. "And that becomes important in terms of understanding mechanisms in play that might be helping to defend against Alzheimer's, or causing what we call *resilience*, where you could have individuals with plaques and tangles apparent in their brains. Before they died, and we did neurocognitive testing, they were intact. How did they do that?"

In the field of gerontology, resilience is a key focus, even though it's far from being fully understood, let alone replicated in pill form. Of greatest interest right now: centenarians who die with razor-sharp minds, displaying little, if any, signs of cognitive decline while alive—and yet their brains, examined upon death, reveal the same telltale plaques and tangles as people with full-blown Alzheimer's. How they've managed to escape Alzheimer's relatively unscathed is a mystery that scientists are still working to unravel.

Inflammation is another area researchers are focusing sharply on, if only because it plays such a central role in aging. Scientists at California's Buck Institute for Research on Aging and at Stanford University—using a tool they developed to measure age-related, chronic inflammation in the human body—compared the "inflammatory ages" of nearly three dozen Italian centenarians with those of people aged fifty to seventy-nine. The centenarians, they found, had inflammatory ages averaging forty years less than their calendar ages.

"We have one outlier: a super-healthy, 105-year-old man who has the immune system of a twenty-five-year-old," says David Furman, an associate professor at the Buck Institute. That's important, Furman says, because inflammation triggers cellular senescence—an otherwise healthy cell's loss of the ability to divide and grow, and a key hallmark of aging and, ultimately, death. "It happens slowly, and it accumulates with time," he says. Inflammation also keeps unhealthy renegade cancer cells alive: "Cells that are cancerous cannot live without inflammation. You fuel them with inflammation, and they grow and metastasize."

If we ever do manage to engineer vastly longer lives, it will be because we've unlocked the secrets of cellular senescence.

IN THE 2009 FILM *MR. NOBODY*, JARED LETO'S TITLE CHARACTER—118-year-old Nemo Nobody, the last surviving mortal on Earth after the human race has attained quasi-immortality—rues the years he feels he squandered. "At my age, the candles cost more than the cake," he laments. "I'm not afraid of dying. I'm afraid I haven't been alive enough."

The age of 150 keeps cropping up, not only in popular culture but on the fringes of some corners of gerontology. It's become trendy to embrace the intoxicating possibilities of a century-and-a-half life span, but don't go gushing to Tom Perls—he's already having difficulty imagining how anyone will eclipse Jeanne Calment's 122 years and 164 days. It's hard enough to get to 105 or 110, says the man who's spent time in the company of Sarah Knauss, who was 119 years and 97 days when she died in 1999 and remains the oldest American who ever lived. Maybe, just maybe, Perls says, someone will live a bit longer than Calment.

"Much beyond that, I just don't see it," he says. "I think 150 is probably unattainable. That's way beyond the pale. Our bodies can only go so far." He takes a decidedly dim view of the British author and biomedical gerontologist Aubrey de Grey, who promotes the view that someone, someday, serendipitously will live to 1,000 simply by benefiting from continuous technological advances over time.

"One of the problems—one of the challenges, if you will—is just how incredibly complex aging is, and all the different things that contribute to that," he says. "You may be able to treat one thing, but your ability to impact the 300 other things is a long shot. And then there's also the big problem that when you tinker with one thing, you may cause a problem with another. The big elephant in the room there is cancer. There's just a very, very strong connection between aging and cancer. And the things that might be good for you in terms of slowing aging might be quite good for increasing your risk of cancer. That's a relationship that's hard to mess with."

In fact, it's all a delicate balance. When I first met Perls, it was May 2020. The coronavirus pandemic was in full fury; much of the world was in lockdown; and I'd reached out to ask about how centenarians were weathering COVID-19. Not well, as it turned out—households were losing the highest limbs on their family trees. People who survived world wars, polio, the Great Depression, and the Holocaust weren't beating COVID-19. There were exceptions, spared by their toughness and genetic good fortune. But globally, the scourge claimed hundreds of centenarians; for Perls, each loss diminishing the planet. "For families, they're the pride and joy, the anchor, the link to the family's history. They're a huge big deal," he lamented at the time. "We truly regard each one of them as a living historical treasure."

Meanwhile, seemingly everywhere we turn, someone is achieving a remarkable age with both body and mind intact. Take Gladys Knight.

No, not *that* Gladys Knight. This one, a long-retired housecleaner in far southeast England, doesn't have any Pips, let alone seven Grammy Awards. But she's a bright and lively 108; back in the day, she loved to dance; and, metaphorically speaking, she's still riding her American namesake's "Midnight Train to Georgia."

For others who've reached or surpassed 106, the journey has been more harrowing. A powerful example is Viola Fletcher, a 110-year-old African American survivor of the Tulsa Race Massacre in 1921, when a mob of white rioters looted and burned more than 1,200 Black-owned homes and businesses, slaughtering as many as 300 and laying waste to a district so thriving and imaginative it had become known as Black Wall Street. On the 100th anniversary of those atrocities, the impact of which still reverberates across society today, Fletcher testified poignantly before Congress about how she can still smell the smoke and hear the screams.

Another Black survivor of Tulsa's horrors, 109-year-old Lessie Randle, told federal lawmakers about what she'd endured: "By the grace of God, I am still here. I have survived to tell this story. I believe that I am still here to share it with you."

Both made it to incredibly advanced ages, but they did so against all odds. As we'll see in the next chapter, the ranks of centenarians—at least in the United States—are a painfully white space.

It's a haunting inequity; one that should trouble us all.

CHAPTER FOUR

THE UNBEARABLE WHITENESS OF BEING A CENTENARIAN

A short drive from my home on the outskirts of Providence, there's a posh retirement community that offers custom-designed flats, including spacious penthouses, for well-heeled elders. "A unique model of gracious senior living," its glossy brochures promise, and they're not kidding. Tasteful oil paintings adorn the walls; there are four dining options, including an alfresco patio; activities include wine tastings of Riesling, Pinot Noir, and other vintages; and residents can treat themselves to massages and facials in the wellness spa.

The Laurelmead Cooperative grabbed headlines a few years ago when, remarkably, it turned out that six of its 200-odd residents were centenarians—an unusually large cluster of people with triple-digit ages living under the same roof. The youngest was 100. The oldest, a former ski champion in her native Switzerland, was 104.

All six were white.

Granted, that may not be all that surprising in a place of privilege that practically screams: *"Pardon me, do you have any Grey Poupon?"*

But US Census Bureau data reflects the same reality: The realm of super-aging, at least in the United States, is an overwhelmingly white space. In fact, only one in ten American centenarians is a person of color.

If that doesn't bother you, it should. Black and brown Americans are at a distinct disadvantage when it comes to longevity. Just think about that. Life is, at its essence, about love and lived experience; and those things require time. White people get more time.

THE AVERAGE LIFE EXPECTANCY FOR BLACKS IN THE UNITED STATES in 2021 was 70.8 years. By contrast, white Americans could expect to live to 76.4. Nearly six years of existence separated the races. That's a lot of life. Think of six-year-olds you have known—they've learned to read, write, and swim; have completed the first grade; and might be preparing to receive their First Communion. It's an unthinkable gap in longevity between races and a glaring inequity we must address.

Experts in demography and racial injustice say it's a consequence of what's known as "weathering theory"—the idea that the health of African Americans begins to deteriorate in early adulthood as a physical consequence of socioeconomic disadvantages that add up and take a toll. It's already evident at the beginning of life, when Black mothers—even wealthy ones—are twice as likely to die of complications from childbirth. And scientists believe it's a factor that keeps a disproportionate number of Black and brown elders from reaching or exceeding 100.

Arline Geronimus, the University of Michigan public health and population researcher who coined the term "weathering," has done pioneering work on the effects of poverty and structural racism on health and longevity. Black women in particular, Geronimus says, age faster and develop chronic diseases such as high blood pressure earlier simply because of the stress of living in a society that discriminates against them.

Geronimus's quest to get to the bottom of the racial gap in aging began when she worked part-time at a school for pregnant teenagers of color in Trenton, New Jersey, while she was a student at Princeton University. She noticed the girls at the school seemed to suffer from chronic illnesses that her mostly white and considerably more affluent fellow Ivy Leaguers rarely had to deal with. That got her wondering about the eroding effects of inescapable poverty, racism, and stress, and the cumulative toll they can take on Black and brown bodies.

Living in a racist society—as Geronimus has found in decades of exhaustive research—compromises Black people's bodies on a cellular level. Ultimately, it leads to poorer health outcomes and shorter longevity. "Accelerated biological aging," Geronimus calls it, and it's one of the primary reasons COVID-19 had such a disproportionate and devastating effect on communities of color, which have higher incidences of hypertension, diabetes, and other chronic conditions. Figures from the US Centers for Disease Control and Prevention lay bare just how harrowing this gap in health and longevity is: African Americans aged eighteen to forty-nine are twice as likely to die of heart disease than whites, and those aged thirty-five to sixty-four are 50 percent more likely to have high blood pressure.

And the inequity goes way beyond illness. Lower-income Americans and, in particular, African Americans are even more likely than whites to be killed in a car crash, the National Safety Council says.

Brian Smedley, a senior fellow in the Office of Race and Equity Research at the Urban Institute think tank, argues that African Americans born in the United States fare more poorly in terms of health than someone born in a developing country such as Jamaica "because of systemic racism here."

"We all know that people of color were hardest hit by COVID and certainly faced higher infection rates and poorer outcomes," Smedley says. "But the lesson of COVID is that it reflected inequities that existed prior to the virus even coming into our world. It was a dual pandemic of racism *and* the viral pandemic. . . . Structural, institutional, and interpersonal racism helps to increase risk for the heavy chronic disease burden that we see in communities of color."

How ironic that, in some gerontological circles, centenarians and supercentenarians are referred to as "black swans"—a reference to Europeans' seventeenth-century belief that the existence of such creatures was impossible. A hundred years later, when black swans turned up for real in western Australia, the term came to define rare and difficult-to-predict events beyond the realm of normal expectation. In a sense, all centenarians, regardless of race and ethnicity, are black swans. But in the United States, at least, people of color who attain triple-digit ages personify the term, if only because of everything they've had to endure to get there.

The life expectancy gap between Blacks and whites in the United States has persisted since 1990, and even though it has narrowed in recent years, all American average life spans still lag well behind those in Europe, according to a 2021 comparison by a Northwestern University team published in the *Proceedings of the National Academy of Sciences*. In the United States, the gap between Black and white life expectancy was narrowing and would have closed in 2036, but progress stalled around 2012 for reasons that still aren't entirely clear. The takeaway, though, is crystal: We're still dying earlier than our friends across the pond. "Even those US populations with the longest life spans—white Americans living in the highest-income areas—experience higher mortality at all ages than Europeans in high-income areas," the researchers warn.

Herlda Senhouse can attest to all of this, and more, even though—as a 113-year-old Black woman—she's clearly an outlier.

"Don't live too fast," she likes to say, and her remarkably long life began slow enough: Born in 1911, one of her childhood chores was to clean her family's oil lamps before electricity reached their home in rural West Virginia. She vividly recalls curling up in bed with a hot iron to help ward off the chill in a house without indoor plumbing; and losing her mother when she was just four and her father when she was only six.

I caught up with her for a delightfully illuminating conversation at her home in an apartment complex for low-income seniors in Wellesley; ironically, one of Massachusetts's wealthiest towns, with more villas and carriage houses per capita than anywhere else in the commonwealth.

Sitting with her couldn't help but remind me of the 1971 Ernest J. Gaines novel *The Autobiography of Miss Jane Pitman*, turned into an Emmy Award–winning, made-for-TV movie in 1974 and starring Cicely Tyson as the fictional Jane. In the movie, Jane narrates her life story, from being a twenty-three-year-old slave at the end of the Civil War to joining the civil rights movement at age 110.

THE FIRST THING YOU NOTICE WHEN YOU STEP INTO HERLDA'S AIRY sixth-floor apartment is the laughter.

I glance around, looking for a TV in a corner on low volume with a sitcom on for background noise. Nope. Those muffled chuckles are coming straight from the supercentenarian herself. Her giggling is lilting, musical, and contagious, and it fills the spaces in our conversation in the loveliest way imaginable. It's soft and soothing and rhythmic—a quiet force of nature, like the breaking of waves on a beach. She may be 113, but by God, this is a woman overflowing with life.

Multiple framed photographs of Barack and Michelle Obama adorn the walls and tabletops of the apartment Herlda has called home for the past forty-plus years. "I've never met them in person, but they sent me pictures. I even have a picture of their dog some-place," she tells me, pointing to a keepsake she especially treasures: a letter from the Obama White House thanking her for her support. "I had a party the day he was elected." (Aside to the nation's forty-fourth POTUS and FLOTUS: Your number one fan is half a century older than you are, and just as quick-witted.)

I'm interviewing her less than twenty-four hours after the death of Britain's Queen Elizabeth at the august age of ninety-six. Although international media are reflecting on the queen's own remark-able longevity and her seventy-year run as the United Kingdom's longest-serving monarch, Herlda was born on February 28, 1911, meaning she was already sixteen when Elizabeth arrived wailing at a world she'd indelibly change.

Herlda rolls her eyes at my opener, a lame attempt at a dad joke: If she'd been born on February 29 instead of February 28, and if it were a leap year, technically she'd be just twenty-eight.

How does she feel, I ask her, to still be going strong at 113? "I have no feelings about it at all," she responds. "It's just the way things are." Deeply devout, yet refreshingly pragmatic, she tells me she's already donated her brain in advance to New England Centenarian Study director Tom Perls's partners at Massachusetts General Hospital. If her cerebrum contains any hidden clues to her extraordinary run, she wants science to figure them out for the rest of us. "I'm going to be cremated, so they might as well put it to good use," she says with a shrug, tapping a temple with an index finger.

Herlda's rules for a long and satisfying life? Live and let live. Don't try to tell people what to do; they want to live their lives as they wish, so let them. If you can't fix something, leave it alone. (That, incidentally, goes for the multiple annoying spam calls that light up her phone during our hour together. Wisely, she lets them go to voicemail.)

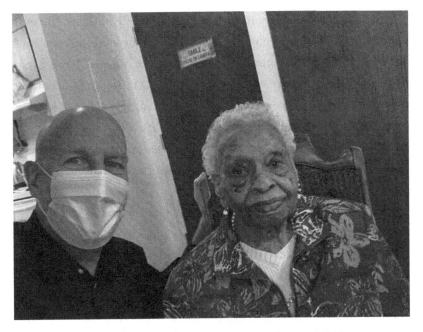

Herlda Senhouse, 113, of Massachusetts with the author. (*William J. Kole*)

Spend any time in the regal presence of this self-confident super-ager, and you'd be struck by her humility and matter-of-factness. She's as bewildered as the rest of us at how she's managed to live so incredibly long with all her faculties intact. "I just take each day as it comes," she says with a shrug. "I've had a journey I never thought I'd ever have. Everything I've got just came to me, and I think it's God's blessing."

Incredibly, and improbably, the days keep coming. But the grand dame is ambivalent when asked how long she'd like to live.

115? 122 and a half? (That's less than a decade away, with the enticement of potential bragging rights as the oldest human who ever lived—even older than Jeanne Calment.) Her logic, a recurring theme as we chat, is as blunt as it is incontrovertible: "If the world was better, I wouldn't mind living that long. But the world is such a mess, I don't want to be here."

Herlda's prime coincided with the height of Jim Crow, the evil patchwork of laws and customs that enforced racial segregation, but she's lived most of her life far north of the Mason-Dixon Line. Even so, the Boston area was riven by racist strife. Mindful of the turbulence I myself grew up in during court-ordered desegregation of Boston's public school system in the 1970s, which touched off mass protests and violent resistance by whites on a scale that at times evoked aspects of South African apartheid, I ask her about her own lived experience as a woman of color.

"I think I've had a pretty good life as a Black woman," she begins. But as we pick apart her past, a less rosy picture emerges. She and her husband, who passed away three decades ago, provided domestic support for a wealthy family in Woburn, Massachusetts, and the couple accompanied the family when they vacationed in Florida. On one occasion, Herlda wanted to buy a hat, but the shopkeeper wouldn't let her try it on first. On another, she and her husband were hassled for sitting in a bus shelter reserved for whites. Microaggressions abounded. Fast-forward to today's grim and seemingly endless George Floyd era of routine and murderous police brutality against Blacks, and she flashes a steely determination: "One day they'll learn we're here, and we're not going anywhere, so they might as well live with us."

If you're getting the impression this woman is laser-focused, and that none of her senses have abandoned her as she advances into her 110s, you'd be right. Sitting across from her, I fumble for my glasses to read some notes, and it occurs to me she isn't wearing any. She's fifty years my senior, yet she needs glasses only for distance, and still gets around using a walker she teasingly calls her Cadillac. What, I ask, is the key to her exceptional longevity?

"You have to keep moving," she says. For her, that means going out to lunch and dinner regularly with her lady friends, though she's not impressed with younger chefs' modern takes on her favorite meals: Recently, she ordered a BLT that came with chicken, avocado, and cranberries. Dessert, strawberry shortcake, was fried Twinkies with vanilla ice cream and a few scarce berries she had trouble locating on her plate because "they went through [the ice cream] on snowshoes." (Her verdict, pronounced with a touch of contempt: "These young chefs really don't know how to cook.") She doesn't like alcohol, though as a younger woman, she vividly recalls a trip to Barbados when she sipped rum and tea, but pauses to clarify: "It was more tea than rum."

Today, her only true vice is the penny slots at the gleaming Encore Casino on the outskirts of Boston. How often does she go to the casino? I ask. "As often as I can," she says, giggling, and mentions proudly that she broke even the last time. She's won as much as $300 in a single sitting. We talk about not overdoing it, so she won't get into trouble, when she interrupts to note: "I can't get into trouble. . . . I don't have much money."

It was at the casino, she says, where a bit of hilarity once played out. A man about your humble author's age was playing the machines next to her, and someone introduced Herlda as a 111-year-old. The man scoffed in disbelief but took a selfie with Herlda, and when he got home, he did a little research. Later, gobsmacked, he contacted one of her friends on Facebook and apologized profusely for doubting her age.

Herlda's greatest comfort is listening to jazz. It's been a lifelong passion, and reviewing her legacy, it's where she's arguably had her greatest impact. Earlier in her life, she founded Boston's Clique Club, a social club of dancers and musicians, to help educate Black students by footing their bills for books and college tuition. She and her husband never had any children of their own, so these were her kids—they and an astonishingly vast network of grandnieces and young friends in their thirties and forties spread over multiple states who treasure time spent with Herlda. (Her nickname is "Auntie," and she's the first to acknowledge it can be confusing: "I was going to church, and everyone would call me Auntie. People said, 'How many nieces and nephews do you have?' And I said, 'Everybody in the church.'")

One of her closest friends is 102, and I ask Herlda what kind of advice she gives her.

"I don't give her advice 'cuz she thinks she knows it all," she says, and chuckles.

What would she tell her friend if she'd listen?

"To be more kind to people. She's kind of harsh."

Maybe she needs more time to mellow, I suggest.

"How much time has she got?" she fires back, then dissolves into a fresh round of those irrepressible giggles.

SOCIETY CLEARLY ISN'T FAVORING BLACK AMERICANS WHO WANT TO live to 100. But if they can make it to eighty-five, an intriguing anomaly suggests they may find the odds of becoming a centenarian swing increasingly in their favor.

Over the past few decades, researchers have demonstrated a fascinating phenomenon that's become known as the "Black-white crossover." Basically, Blacks who reach eighty-five in good shape have demonstrated their survival prowess, and at that point, their ability to go on to 100 or older is demonstrably better than that of their white counterparts. Some demographers question it, but Perls finds it plausible.

Blacks in their mid-eighties and older "have kind of gotten over this hump, and to get there, they had to be in amazing shape to fight all the problems of structural racism," Perls tells me. "If they've gotten to that point, they really have demonstrated this increased ability to age slowly and get to a very old age. And that makes them a different group than whites of the same age."

A notable 2008 Georgia State University study of supercentenarians bore that out. It identified 355 individuals aged 110
or older whose ages could be verified, creating the first reliable
American dataset for this population group. "I found it intriguing
that . . . nine of the eleven former Confederate states of America
had as their all-time oldest verified person an African American,"
wrote lead researcher Robert Douglas Young. At the time Young
was studying the phenomenon, three of the four oldest living
Americans were Black.

Among those who've beaten the odds: Wendy McCrae-Owoeye's
grandmother, who lived to 104.

McRae-Owoeye, an assistant vice president for human resources
at Providence College, identifies as biracial. Her grandmother, a
member of the Cherokee Nation who was partly white, grew up on a
tribal reservation in Georgia, enduring racism in a household dominated by a spiteful stepmother who disliked her dark complexion.
Sent off to boarding school, she fell in love with a handsome multiracial young man, and the couple eloped, eventually settling in Rhode
Island. They raised a family through the turbulence of entrenched
discrimination and racial injustice that rocked even their adoptive
northern state, once dubbed "the Mississippi of New England" partly
because of Ku Klux Klan activity in now-tony Newport. Somehow, it
didn't diminish her life span.

Given the genes McCrae-Owoeye likely inherited from her family's 104-year-old matriarch, does the now fifty-eight-year-old expect
to live to 100 herself?

"I hope not," she says, recalling "The Talk" she's had to give her
twenty-two-year-old son: If the police stop you, put your hands in the
air, never in your pockets. If you're pulled over, keep your hands right
on the top of the dashboard, don't flinch, don't move. When he was
four and shoplifted a pack of gum, she first marched him back to the
store to return it; then headed straight to the nearest police station to

have him placed in a cell for a few minutes. The good-natured desk sergeant thought it was cute and played along, but she's dead serious about what could happen to her son during a traffic stop, now that he's an adult Black male.

I thought about this the other evening as I was riding in my brother's SUV and he was pulled over for a license plate bulb the officer deemed a little too dim. It was a bullshit stop, and we did little to conceal our annoyance. In that moment, my Black friends' experiences came tumbling back to my mind, and I realized anew how expressing irritation at the police without worrying in the slightest about potentially deadly pushback is the unique prerogative of the white male. As the deferential young officer politely let us off with a warning, my brother and I talked about how the stop might have gone differently had we been two Black men wandering the predominantly white suburbs where we grew up. A backup unit likely would have been called, and we'd have been asked to get out of the car; the prelude to God knows what, with or without any back talk. Little wonder a new Yale study finds that stress makes us age faster, speeds up our biological clocks, and shortens our life spans.

Entrenched hatred and racism aren't the only problems that give McCrae-Owoeye pause. She's also troubled by economic inequities and the devastating effects of climate change. "There are just so many major concerns. So, I mean, if my destiny is to live to be 100, then I hope it's a productive 100 years. But if it's a situation where there's pain and turmoil, I don't want to be here."

Setting aside a favorable family history, studies show you're a prime candidate for 100 if you've got a good socioeconomic status at midlife, you're a nonsmoker, you eat cleanly, and you exercise regularly. But here's the catch: For much of the world, fresh, healthy food, time to exercise, and access to preventive health care are luxuries.

"Not only are good food, time to exercise, and access to reasonable health care in short supply in many parts of the world, but they're in short supply in many parts of the US," says Beth Truesdale, a sociologist focused on inequities in aging and work at the W.E. Upjohn Institute for Employment Research in Kalamazoo, Michigan.

Americans, she notes, tend to think rather simplistically about individual choices around diet and exercise, assuming everyone at least has the power to move their bodies and decide what to eat. But, of course, it's never that simple.

"If you think it's an easy personal choice to eat healthy food, maybe that's because you can afford fresh, healthy food, and maybe you have access to be able to buy good food locally. You have the time and the energy to prepare healthy food," Truesdale tells me. "Likewise, if you think it's an easy personal choice to get daily exercise, that everybody can exercise, maybe that's because you live in a safe neighborhood for walking, for jogging. Maybe you have some nearby parks. You have a place to go for recreation. Maybe you can afford to pay something for your exercise. I'm not even talking here about fancy gym memberships, but to be able to buy a good pair of shoes to go for long walks, and to have the time to be able to exercise and to take care of yourself in that way. All these things are super unequal in the US and around the world."

Truesdale says her research bears solemn witness to the veracity of Geronimus's weathering theory: "It's 100 percent absolutely real."

"White people tend to live so much longer than Black people on average, and rich people tend to live so much longer than poor people on average," she says. "We have a huge amount of evidence that racism exists at the individual level, at the cultural level, and at the structural level. Racism that you encounter from people giving you a hard time in daily life is the individual level. It goes right through to the structural level: If you're Black, your grandparents probably didn't have wealth they passed down to your parents, and which your parents are passing down to you. The places where your parents, your grandparents lived are going to be fundamentally different than the places where many white people's parents and grandparents lived. The resources today's generations have to be able to age well are completely different. That's hugely important."

Much of Truesdale's research has examined the effects of toxic stress on aging bodies—and if anyone in American society is hammered relentlessly by stress, it's people of color.

"We have huge amounts of evidence that the racism that you experience in the US and elsewhere is very stressful. We've come to really understand how toxic stress—the kind of stress that doesn't go away, that you can't do anything about—affects all the body systems," she says. "Those of us who live pretty cushy lives often think stress is like, 'Oh, I've got a work deadline.' But I have resources I can use to encounter that stress and meet the demand. That's not necessarily bad for my health. But the kind of stress that comes from, 'There's no way I can pay the rent; I'm going to get evicted'—the kind of stress that comes from, 'I cannot stretch the budget to the end of the month, and somebody is going to have to eat less, or less well, than I wish they could'—those sorts of stress really get to the body. That's a sort of socioeconomic piece, but then there's also the racism piece. In the US, those two things are often quite tightly intertwined, but they're not the same. Both matter. You can't separate it out and say it's either one or the other."

And America doesn't have a monopoly on misery. Outside the United States, toxic stress and diminished life expectancy are grim and daily realities for billions.

Stress affects us all right down to the cellular level, says Dr. Martin Picard of Columbia University, an expert in what's become known as mitochondrial psychobiology. "Stress, as we experience it, triggers a release of hormones. Stress is damaging because it takes energy away from the longevity-promoting operations in the cells.

It diverts resources away from those things that keep the organism healthy," Picard tells me. He likens a body operating on high alert because of stress to a government investing multiple billions in its army and mere pennies on health care or infrastructure.

Esther Duflo and Abhijit Banerjee of the Massachusetts Institute of Technology, whose anti-poverty research won them the 2019 Nobel Memorial Prize in Economic Sciences, have extensively documented the life-shortening effects of lacking the basics. "When the poor come under economic stress, their form of 'insurance' is often eating less or taking their children out of school," they write in a seminal study. And as we'll see, education—especially a college education—is a key to longevity.

IF ALL THIS IS TRUE, HOW DO WE EXPLAIN PEOPLE LIKE 110-YEAR-old Viola Fletcher, whom we met in chapter 3? She didn't have an opportunity to continue her schooling past the fourth grade and survived the 1921 Tulsa Race Massacre, one of the worst incidents of racial violence in US history, yet she lived deep into her 100s. What stress could be more toxic than seeing your neighbors murdered in cold blood and their homes and businesses burned to the ground?

A century later, Tulsa's pain remains palpable, and artists across the vast musical spectrum are still composing powerful works of commemoration and catharsis.

One is *Fire in Little Africa*, a hip-hop album released by Motown Records' Black Forum label that executive producer Stevie Johnson describes as "a communal undoing of trauma . . . the rose that grows out of the concrete."

Another is *Pity These Ashes, Pity This Dust*, an operatic piece staged on the centennial of the slaughter by a trio of Harlem performing arts and chamber music groups. "The story of African Americans in this country is a story of survival," composer Adolphus Hailstork says.

World War II epitomized the depths of human cruelty and suffering. Yet two of America's oldest male supercentenarians, both of whom left us in 2022, endured the horrors of its battlefields while serving in racially segregated units, only to return to a homeland where dark-skinned war heroes—and anyone else with the misfortune to have been born Black in the Jim Crow era—were treated *at best* as "separate but equal." Baltimore native Ezra Edward Hill Sr., who witnessed the invasion of Normandy and was injured in combat, returned to a United States that was still years away from birthing the modern civil rights movement. Against all odds, he lived to 111.

Lawrence Brooks of New Orleans served as a private in the US Army's mostly Black 91st Engineer Battalion. Born in 1909 to a sharecropper couple, he was one of fifteen children. Drafted within weeks of the Japanese attack on Pearl Harbor into a military that was still racially segregated, he helped build roads and bridges while stationed in Australia, New Guinea, and the Philippines. "We had our tents, and the whites had their tents," Brooks told the *Military Times*. He especially enjoyed his time in Australia, where Black soldiers were readily accepted, recalling: "I was treated so much better in Australia than I was (at home) by my own white people." He longed to study after the war, but back in the United States, he and other decorated Black war veterans routinely were denied benefits under the GI Bill, which was supposed to provide all returning servicemen with an education, low-interest bank loans, unemployment allowances, job placement assistance, and a reduced down payment for a house. If it was any consolation, he vastly outlived the bureaucrats who stamped "REJECTED" on that paperwork, soldiering on to the venerable and incredible age of 112.

Adding insult to injury, even Hollywood long ignored the bravery and sacrifice of soldiers of color in World War II. That didn't change until 2008, when Spike Lee's groundbreaking *Miracle at St. Anna*—based on James McBride's 2002 novel of the same name—became the first major motion picture to feature Black conscripts in a notoriously white genre.

World War II's humiliations and injustices, and Tulsa's wanton bloodletting, inflicted the kind of next-level stress most of us will never experience. How, then, does someone like a Fletcher or a Brooks endure such horrors and go on to live to 108 or 112?

Truesdale explains: "As humans, we're really bad at thinking about probability. For example, if you don't smoke, that doesn't guarantee that you'll live to 100, but it makes it more likely. Everything puts a little finger on the scale. Everything provides a little boost. Not smoking gives you a little bit of a boost. Not being poor gives you a bit of a boost. Having the resources to be able to eat well gives you a bit of a boost. All these things weigh on the scale in some way or another, but they don't guarantee anything. And so, while Black people are more likely to die younger in the US than white people are, you'll have exceptions on both sides. And while rich people are likely to live longer than poor people on average, and the gaps are big, you have exceptions. And because the exceptions are often so notable, we think it must not matter—you must be able to live long no matter what.

"We see the eighty-year-old yoga teacher, and we think, 'Oh, well, we just need to keep working longer. That's how you stay active.' Of course, it doesn't really work like that for many, many people. It *does* work like that for *some* small number of people. Great for them. But it doesn't work like that for everyone, and the trends are in the opposite direction."

Ironically, the seminal research that laid bare the brutal effects of job stress began with a study of white people. In a landmark 2015 study, Princeton economists Anne Case and Nobel laureate Angus Deaton showed that death rates among white, middle-aged Americans were rising—bucking decades of decline—not because of heart disease or diabetes, but for largely self-inflicted reasons:

suicide, alcohol-induced liver disease, and overdoses of prescription opiates.

Initially, a clear-cut cause of this self-destruction eluded them. But as the husband-and-wife team investigated, they noticed these white, non-Hispanic men and women who were dying early had something in common: They lacked a college degree, which meant reduced social and economic mobility. Translation: Those of us who find ourselves stuck at a certain rung on the economic ladder generally don't live as long as those with the resources to buy a home or move to a place with cleaner air and water and better schools and other amenities. Over the past generation or so, Case and Deaton found that white people with less than a bachelor's degree no longer can assume they'll be better off than their parents, which was the assumption of the previous generation. Their blunt takeaway: "Without a four-year college diploma, it is increasingly difficult to build a meaningful and successful life in the United States." People with some college, and those earning a good living through a skilled trade, do better than those who don't advance their educations beyond high school—but it's those with the sheepskins who enjoy the most economic security, greatest earning power, and better overall health.

Subsequent research shows the lack of a college degree corresponds to greater mortality across all racial and ethnic groups, not just whites. That makes this a problem that's bigger than the white working class. It's a problem for Americans at large.

And something else is going on. Until the early 2010s, mortality rates among Blacks and Latinos were improving, incrementally closing the gap between whites and non-whites in terms of life expectancy. Black and Latino mortality is climbing again, and the gap between them and whites remains large and persistent. Throughout their life spans, Black Americans have much higher mortality rates and much worse health than whites do, and by pretty much every measure. It's a huge inequity.

In the late 1970s and early 1980s, I put myself through college by working a series of blue-collar jobs, all for minimum wage. I pumped gas; worked as a laborer for a stonemason, mixing mortar and hauling bricks and concrete blocks until my back needed icing; stood for hours on end doing grunt work in a print shop; and drove a truck around three states for a ceramics distributor. I learned not only to acknowledge my white male privilege—for me, the grind of working hard for meager pay was just for a season—but to value and respect the blood, sweat, and tears that many people shed daily throughout their lifetimes to feed themselves and their kids, and position them to achieve their own dreams.

What stuck with me since is how their plight introduces yet more disturbing inequity into the calculus of who lives the longest. Money can't buy you love, but apparently, it can help you lease more life. How is that fair?

America in the mid-2020s ought to be a place of unrivaled opportunity. Instead, too many are working two or more jobs just to survive. Truesdale, whose lifework has involved keeping painfully close tabs on these trends, sees a connection between economic struggle and diminished life span.

"We make those things harder by the way that we set up work," she tells me. A prime example: the millions of Americans who do shift work. Some don't know their schedule until two days in advance; others have to close up shop at night, only to reopen a few hours later in the morning. "All that takes a physical toll. The control you have over your time is really impactful on your health. As a society, we've decided that we're going to allow employers to impose those sorts of last-minute and unsustainable kinds of schedules on workers. As a society, we could decide to do something about that."

Other things we could do something about: not rushing to judgment about people who are less fit (read: fatter) or active than some of us might be. If you're within walking, or even easy driving, distance of a grocery store, count yourself fortunate, because millions of Americans live in food deserts bereft of easy access to the basics. Having access to a good grocery store won't guarantee you'll live to 100, any more than not having access to one means you'll die young, but it puts that finger back on the scale.

Caitlin Daniel, a sociologist at the University of California, Berkeley, has done intriguing research into why low-income parents tend to buy less healthy food for their children than higher-income parents do. Beyond issues of cost, access, food deserts, and the time and energy it takes to prepare healthy meals without a stable work schedule, Daniel interviewed low-income parents at grocery stores and asked what they were buying and why. Higher-income parents, she discovered, can afford to buy broccoli twenty times—even if their children refuse to eat it nineteen times and it gets tossed in the trash—to teach them to eventually appreciate and consume food that's good for them. Lower-income parents, by contrast, can't afford to waste food, so they buy something less nutritious they know their kids will eat.

It's the same set of realities that prompts a single parent working two jobs to resort to a fast-food drive-thru, if only because it's cheap and she knows her kids will eat it. Millions of Americans make these decisions every day—not necessarily because they want to, but because it's an affordable path of least resistance. In the long term, it undermines their health. And the way people of privilege view these patterns is unhelpful, if not downright racist.

Asked what we need to do to respond to all of this, Truesdale gives a long pause, and then draws a connection straight to politics. If we're going to make meaningful steps toward improving Americans' health and leveling the playing field in terms of who among us has a shot at a triple-digit life, she contends, it's going to take a functioning democracy that responds to the needs of ordinary citizens. "And we're in a situation right at the moment where that's not a guarantee," she says. "Politics produces policy. Policies have downstream consequences for people's health."

What's at stake: even wider gaps in longevity between the rich and the poor.

For instance, researchers have found that in the United States, men in the top 25 percent in income at age forty can expect to live to about eighty-seven on average. Men in the bottom 25 percent of wage-earners? Ten years less. And that troubling income/longevity gap is similar, if somewhat smaller, for women. It is, arguably, the most egregious inequality of all: The rich get more time.

For those who are morally offended and demand change, sociologists and think tanks tick off some practical options. For starters, raise the income of people in the bottom half through a higher federal minimum wage. Provide a more robust safety net for people who have disabilities and those who are out of work. Give workers a greater voice, partly by reviving labor unions, which, until a surprising resurgence in the early 2020s, had unspooled badly over the previous few decades. And find ways to help more people enjoy the life span benefits of a college degree, which go beyond someone's bank account. Education helps you speak up for yourself. People who have college educations are more likely to be taken seriously at a doctor's office, and to take care of their own health. They're also less likely to smoke than people who lack a degree.

Another emerging advantage wealthy whites hold over people of color with fewer resources: It's easier for them to move away from areas imperiled by the effects of climate change.

Researchers have found that people working in hot conditions—think agriculture, construction, landscaping—suffer poorer health and live shorter lives than those with jobs in air-conditioned buildings. It's an issue that OSHA, the Occupational Safety and Health Administration, is attempting to address. But the federal agency is accustomed to addressing more clear and present workplace dangers, such as machines capable of chopping off a worker's arm. Responding to the slightly more abstract effects of climate change as a workplace threat is difficult enough, and it gets even trickier when you add the aging piece. Older workers are more susceptible to the heat. How will a fifty-five-year-old construction worker fare when framing a building in temperatures reaching 110 degrees Fahrenheit? It was no sweat, comparatively speaking, when that worker was twenty-five and temperatures didn't get much hotter than 90 degrees.

Dealing with an unfavorable climate—especially when we're older—is an age-old struggle. Even Hippocrates noticed. Four centuries before Christ, he wrote of people living in humid and marshy wetlands:

> The children are particularly subject to hernia, and adults to varices and ulcers on their legs, so that persons with such constitutions cannot be long-lived, but before the usual period they fall into a state of premature old age.

IF ALL THESE TRENDS CONTINUE, WHITE CENTENARIANS—THROUGH no fault of their own—risk widening the rift between the races merely by existing.

Consider this: The Census Bureau projects that in just a little more than two decades from now, in 2045, the United States will become a "minority white" nation. Whites will comprise 49.7 percent of the population; Hispanics, 24.6 percent; Blacks, 13.1 percent; and Asians, 7.9 percent. People identifying as multiracial will make up the remaining 3.8 percent. Translation: more people of color with diminished life spans watching their white neighbors live appreciably longer.

Marcella Alsan is a Harvard physician and economist who's been investigating the roles that legacies of discrimination and resulting mistrust play in perpetuating racial disparities in health. The COVID pandemic, she says, threw that inequity into sharp relief. A disproportionate number of Black and brown people couldn't work from home because of their jobs in health care, the building trades, or grocery stores. Because they were far more likely than whites to lack health insurance and paid sick leave, their exposure to the virus was greater—too often with deadly consequences—and lifesaving vaccines weren't as accessible to them as they were in affluent white communities. For researchers like Alsan, it all adds up to an indictment.

"Health disparities in the United States are profound," she says. "I think physicians and economists are still struggling to understand the role that structural racism has played in the distribution of resources and the outcomes of illness or health."

So, how do we narrow that gap? Could our very life spans threaten to inflame the divide between the planet's haves and have-nots? So far, answers have eluded even our greatest thinkers—minds like MIT's Duflo and Banerjee. "No one knows how to transform Kenya into South Korea," the academic power couple concedes in a commentary for *Foreign Affairs*.

That brings us back full circle to 70.8—the average life expectancy for a Black American. It turns out that very number, 70.8, resurfaces with overtones of inequity in the medical literature.

When the National Health Interview Survey, the data-collection program within the CDC, asked people how they rated their own health and that of their families, 70.8 percent of non-Hispanic whites assessed it as excellent or very good. Hispanics and non-Hispanic Blacks trailed significantly, at 57.8 percent and 56.9 percent, respectively.

So much for life being whatever we make of it.

Like it or not, we're all hurtling collectively into a rapidly aging world that can't shake its obsession with youngness. What happens when the coming flood of extreme longevity collides with the heady and alluring waters of the mythical yet enduring Fountain of Youth?

I've covered presidents, prime ministers, and popes, and Herlda Senhouoc is far and away one of the coolest people I've ever met in more than four decades as a journalist. Will younger generations agree—especially if all of us in the human collective, young and old, find ourselves competing for resources and influence in a society where ageism is rampant?

Forgive the cliché, but it's true: Time really will tell.

CHAPTER FIVE

GROWING OLD IN A YOUTH-OBSESSED, AGEIST SOCIETY

It's three in the morning and I'm still awake, staring at the ceiling again, trying in vain to pinpoint the moment I became yesterday's man.

For a very long time, I was a go-to guy, jumping on planes to cover political upheaval on four continents; summits that gathered world leaders; and acts both of terror and of God. At times, it was too much—I couldn't even do my laundry before boomeranging back out to the next far-flung assignment. It was exhausting and, I'm not going to lie, exhilarating.

Lately, though, in the twilight of a distinctive and satisfying forty-year journalism career—still at the top of my game and with three foreign languages in my arsenal—the opportunities are gone. No one's ever said anything. No one ever would. But suddenly there's an early retirement option on the table, and in the adrenaline-rush world of the twenty-four-hour news cycle, where the lines between perception and reality frequently blur, I find myself wondering something many late-career employees like me have asked themselves: Am I past my sell-by date? How could I be when Dr. Jane Goodall is ninety and working like never before?

As I anguish over whether to stay or exit early, at least I still have agency. It'll be my decision alone; no one will make it for me. Lisa LaFlamme, one of North America's best-known broadcasters, can't say the same.

FEW POP CULTURE ICONS ARE AS UBIQUITOUS OR INSTANTLY RECOG-nizable as Wendy, the stylized, freckled face of the eponymous fast-food chain. So, when the mascot's trademark pigtails went gray for a day in the company's Canadian restaurants, it touched off a social media sensation.

Pretty much everyone in Canada knew exactly what was up, even without reading the burger giant's tweet: "Because a star is a star regardless of hair color." TV viewers across all ten provinces and three territories have been up in arms over the abrupt August 2022 dismissal of LaFlamme, a hugely popular network news anchor. The reason for her firing wasn't fabricating the news or bias or insubordi-nation or any other legitimate cause. Instead, the fifty-nine-year-old broadcast journalist, as much a household name in Canada as Diane Sawyer is in the United States, says Bell Media let her go after thirty-five years at CTV News because—*quelle horreur!*—she'd let her hair go naturally gray.

LaFlamme says she stopped dyeing her hair during the COVID-19 pandemic, when it was risky to see her stylist and she found herself spraying her roots before going on the air. In a 2020 year-end broad-cast, she told viewers: "Why bother? I'm going gray. Honestly, if I had known the lockdown could be so liberating on that front, I would have done it a lot sooner." Many viewers, especially older women, applauded LaFlamme—but not her employer. After *The Globe and Mail* newspaper reported a CTV executive had openly questioned her decision to let her hair naturally gray, angry cries of age discrimination ensued.

"The news business is one of the most age discriminatory businesses—particularly TV, but all the rest of journalism as well," says Sonni Efron, a longtime journalist for the *Los Angeles Times* and a past president and chief operating officer of the National Press Foundation in Washington, DC.

Age discrimination in general "is so pervasive we don't even notice it," adds Debra Whitman, executive vice president and chief public policy officer at AARP. Her organization regularly asks people aged sixty-five and older if they've seen or personally experienced ageism; three in four respond with an emphatic, if embittered, yes. And just as the pandemic exposed and rattled the fault lines around entrenched racism, it inflamed age discrimination. "There were conversations about having to be under a certain age in order to get access to life support," Whitman says. "There were conversations about how older people should just sacrifice themselves for the good of the economy and their grandchildren."

LaFlamme's ordeal underscores this reality about extreme aging, or really, aging on any scale: We're all growing older in a culture that worships youth far more than it reveres elders. If many of us are destined to be 100, how are we going to experience that in a society that values the young over the old? Our species obsessed over the mythical Fountain of Youth long before Spanish explorer Ponce de Leon's famed quest to find it in the early 1500s.

I don't know about you, but I've always found a loveliness and an elegance to a beautiful, silver-haired woman. (Full disclosure: I'm married to one, and she's spirited and girlish and the life of every party.) "White hair is a crown of glory," the Book of Proverbs insists, so why should anyone be ashamed of it?

Goodall certainly isn't. Her signature ponytail—once blond, now silver—is her trademark. Chronological age be damned: She's one of the most youthful people I've ever had the privilege of interviewing. (She opened a recent appearance in Denver by hooting and panting like a chimp, then telling the crowd: "That simply means, 'This is me—this is Jane.'") And she's still going strong, working harder now than she did as a younger woman, with zero intention of stopping. Her drive and determination underscore how, for some, ninety is the new sixty.

We caught up with her in chapter 1, and we'll visit with her again in chapter 10. Meanwhile, let's take a hard look at the widening gap between the virtues of youth and extreme old age in twenty-first-century culture.

In the 1985 Ron Howard movie *Cocoon*, a group of seniors sneaks into a swimming pool, where they find themselves suddenly infused with youthful vigor. "I feel tremendous! I feel ready to take on the world!" one of them bellows between cannonballs. "We'll never be sick, we won't get any older, and we won't ever die," marvels another. There's just one very big problem: It's only happening because alien cocoons are at the bottom of the deep end. It's an entertaining film, but one with a troubling takeaway—at a certain age, only an encounter with the supernatural can make us feel young again, and only a journey to a distant planet where no one ever grows old can keep us that way. As one senior citizen told the *Los Angeles Times*: "So that's the ultimate solution to the problems of the elderly: Put them on a spaceship and send them to Mars."

You can decide for yourself if *Cocoon* is ageist, but this much is clear: Ageism abounds. Don't just take my word for it: A 2021 report by the World Health Organization warns that age discrimination already is damaging our health and well-being. That raises a troubling question: What will happen when our world is populated by so many more exceptionally old people than ever before?

"For older people, ageism is associated with a shorter life span, poorer physical and mental health, slower recovery from disability, and cognitive decline," the WHO cautions. "Ageism reduces older people's quality of life, increases their social isolation and loneliness (both of which are associated with serious health problems), restricts their ability to express their sexuality, and may increase the risk of violence and abuse against older people."

Why does all that matter? Because Americans, particularly baby boomers, are living and working longer, says William Beach, until recently commissioner of the US Bureau of Labor Statistics. Those aged seventy and up who are participating in the labor force currently amount to 9 percent, Beach says, and it's expected to rise to about 16 percent by 2035. "The baby boom generation is the healthiest and wealthiest ever to walk the face of the Earth," he says. But that's in general, he hastens to add, noting many won't have a choice but to keep working, if only because their retirement savings are so paltry. The median amount of money Americans have stashed away for when they eventually stop working is a woefully insufficient $30,000. "We're now looking at a reality of a lot of older people working," Beach says. "Maybe they choose to work, but so often, they need the money."

And the very notion of retirement itself is essentially a post–World War II phenomenon. The first pension paid out in the United States was issued by an insurance company in 1879. Those who retired before, say, 1860 were independently wealthy Benjamin Franklin types. It's amazing to realize that one of America's most famous inventors, scientists, statesmen, printers, publishers, and founding fathers made it all the way to eighty-four, considering his extracurricular activities. (Would *you* fly a kite in a thunderstorm?) Franklin, though, was a man of many modifiers, and chief among those was "rich." Practically penniless in his early days, the self-made man whose image adorns the $100 bill was his era's equivalent of a multimillionaire. Unlike me, he didn't have to crunch the numbers to see if he could afford to retire. He simply slowed down.

"If you went back three generations, you'd find retirement wasn't as common, and four generations ago, it wasn't common at all," Beach says. "People who retired were people with assets; otherwise, men and women lived their lives using their bodies primarily as the tool of production." Before industrialization, when nearly all of us worked in agriculture, many men developed major muscular, skeletal, and vascular problems by the time they were forty. If they lived that long, they had a good chance of making it to fifty-five, Beach says, "and that's about it. Your last few years might be spent in poverty because most people were poor. Their families were poor. They didn't have assets to look after the people who were older."

Just to underscore what a crapshoot eighteenth-century life expectancy was, consider the renowned English historian, writer, and parliamentarian Edward Gibbon. The first of six volumes that comprised his most acclaimed work, *The History of the Decline and Fall of the Roman Empire*, was published in 1776—the same year that America as an independent nation was born. Incredibly, this Edward was the *sixth* Edward Gibbon to be born to his parents, Edward and Judith Gibbon, who wearily kept naming their boys Edward and watching them die in infancy.

The Gibbons put their trust in doctors, just as we do today. But is that trust misplaced?

Ageism is agonizingly well documented among doctors, nurses, and other health care professionals. In fact, it's become an entrenched part of the equation to determine who gets the most effective (read: expensive) treatment. But as significantly more of us live to 100 and beyond, we need to rethink how we apply our most cutting-edge and costly medical care. At some point, a centenarian is going to want a heart or a kidney. If their underlying health is sound and their prognosis is good, who are we to deny them?

As our planet ages, society is increasingly preoccupied with demanding that older people be treated with dignity and respect.

Elders, once revered, increasingly are reviled. Pulitzer Prize–winning gerontologist Robert Butler coined the term "ageism" in 1969, and sadly, systematic stereotyping and discrimination based on age never gets old.

Pope Francis is among the latest to wade into this complicated conversation. It's not hard to understand why: Slowed by frailty and physical decline as he approaches ninety, the Argentinian-born pontiff has been using a wheelchair and clutching at the arms of his aides, and he's even broached the possibility of following his predecessor, Benedict XVI, into what would pass as early retirement for an octogenarian pope. On a recent pilgrimage to western Canada, Francis urged humanity to construct "a future in which the elderly are not cast aside because, from a 'practical' standpoint, they are no longer useful . . . a future that is not indifferent to the need of the aged to be cared for and listened to."

It's a refrain the pope repeatedly has emphasized. In *On Heaven and Earth*, a 2010 book that preceded his papacy, the then-cardinal Jorge Bergoglio likened ignoring older people's health care needs to "covert euthanasia." Much more recently, Francis has been invoking extreme longevity in the Bible, including our friend Methuselah, and musing over the human condition in the passing of time. "When you return home and there is a grandfather or grandmother who is perhaps no longer lucid or, I don't know, has lost some of their ability to speak, and you stay with him or with her, you are 'wasting time,' but this 'waste of time' strengthens the human family," the pontiff says. "Do you know how to waste time with grandparents, with the elderly? . . . The elderly have much to teach us about the meaning of life."

That's a mellow enough message, but make no mistake: Francis calls down fire and brimstone on those who are indifferent, or worse, to the needs of the aged. After taking over from Benedict XVI when the Pope Emeritus retired in 2013, Francis condemned what he called a "throwaway culture" that treats elders like trash.

For many employers, it makes perfect sense, at least as far as the bottom line is concerned. Sociologist Beth Truesdale, whom we met in chapter 4, coedited *Overtime: America's Aging Workforce and the Future of Working Longer.* The book includes an interview with Henry, a New York City bartender in his early seventies who loves his job; the people, the performance. He's exceptionally good at it, and let's be real: Bartenders are essential workers. They're like social workers or priests and pastors; they listen, and they take our confessions. Henry's only sin: his age. When he had to look for a new gig, the jobs tap abruptly ran dry. "Who's going to hire the sixty-year-old when you can have a cute twenty-five-year-old?" Truesdale asks rhetorically.

It's blatantly illegal. But, maddeningly, it's almost impossible to prove. "Less than 10 percent of age discrimination claims are settled in favor of claimants, and most of them are just dismissed," says Ruth Finkelstein, executive director of the Brookdale Center for Healthy Aging at City University of New York.

Raymond Peeler, associate legal counsel for the federal Equal Employment Opportunity Commission, explains why: "It's rare that we have a smoking gun." Of the 60,000 complaints it reviews annually, the EEOC picks its battles, intervening with a lawsuit in only about 200 cases a year in instances where the agency thinks it can make a difference, Peeler tells me. Private attorneys go after many others, but tens of thousands of Americans who are convinced they've been screwed out of a job never get their day in court.

Those who do wait months or years for justice, says AARP's chief litigator, Bill Rivera: "It's not for the faint of heart."

And despite the fact that people fifty and older are pumping more than $8 trillion a year into the US economy—collectively powering a turbocharged engine that's forecast to rev to $12.6 trillion by 2030 and an astounding $28.2 trillion by 2050—most companies don't include age in their diversity, equity, and inclusion programs.

The federal Age Discrimination in Employment Act, or ADEA, was enacted in 1967, and it covers Americans aged forty and up. (It badly needs updating: Experts note wryly that in some parts of the economy, such as in Silicon Valley, where youth is especially prized, you can find yourself marginalized in your thirties.) Older applicants beware: Job ads can contain coded messages that bely a company's preference for younger workers: "We're seeking digital natives," or, "new college graduates are encouraged to apply."

In 2009, a US Supreme Court decision severely eroded age discrimination protections in employment by making it much easier for employers to fire or demote workers because of their age. Older employees who go to court to challenge their dismissals or demotions now must meet a higher burden of proof.

Jack Gross, a Des Moines, Iowa, insurance company executive, had sued after he was demoted in his mid-fifties. Gross's job performance was in the top 5 percent at FBL Financial Services, and he'd received steady promotions and increased job responsibilities—until he became a man of a certain age, and key tasks were given to a much younger coworker. When the case reached the Supreme Court, it ruled 5–4 against Gross, gutting ADEA in the process. Prior to the high court's ruling, someone like Gross only had to establish that age played a *significant* role in a discriminatory employment action. Now, a plaintiff has to prove that age was the *deciding* factor. It's a legal standard substantially higher than what the law requires for any other type of discrimination—including cases involving race, sex, or religion—and lawyers say it's nearly impossible to meet.

The court's conservative majority—led by Justice Clarence Thomas and joined by Chief Justice John G. Roberts Jr. and Justices Antonin Scalia, Anthony M. Kennedy, and Samuel A. Alito Jr.—said workers bear the full burden of proving that age was the motivating factor in their demotion or dismissal. Employers, of course, never announce they're discriminating against someone because of age. Justice John Paul Stevens wrote a fiery dissent, denouncing the ruling as "especially irresponsible." A decade and a half later, it's had a chilling effect: Winning an age discrimination lawsuit is rare.

Congress has been trying to restore some of those lost protections. One bill that passed the House with broad bipartisan support would allow affected workers to pursue so-called mixed motive claims—allegations of age discrimination against employers who hide behind other factors such as a reorganization or a downsizing. Another, also broadly supported by House Democrats and Republicans, would make it illegal to ask applicants for their birth dates.

But as legislative remedies languish, the abuses heaped upon older workers keep piling up.

In a blockbuster investigation for *ProPublica* that was copublished in 2018 with *Mother Jones*, journalist Peter Gosselin unmasked rampant and brazen age discrimination perpetrated by IBM against older employees. And it's not just IBM. "Fifty-six percent of those who enter their 50s employed full-time in stable jobs are laid off at least once or leave their jobs under financially damaging circumstances that suggest involuntary decisions," Gosselin says. Nine in ten of those, he adds, take an earnings hit from which they'll never recover—even if they're fortunate enough to find a new job, which is far from a given—meaning they'll eventually retire without the nest eggs they'd planned to live on.

Reality check: No matter how old you are, if you apply online for a job, artificial intelligence will suss out your age. And if it's not optimal, good luck getting an interview. AI is ageist, a recent World Health Organization analysis found, concluding that the algorithms powering it tend to not represent the oldest of us; rather, it favors younger individuals.

I can't help but wonder if that explains the crickets that greeted my applications for positions at other leading media outlets virtually identical to the job I've been doing for a decade. To give myself a fighting chance, I carefully scrubbed my résumé to omit any dates that would make my age obvious, yet I never even got an interview. Did AI read between the lines and refuse to advance my candidacy? I'll never know, and if you're my age and find yourself in a similar situation, neither will you.

Skeptical? Try this experiment: Spend a little time clicking around Glassdoor (https://www.glassdoor.com/index.htm), a website where people post anonymous and unvarnished reviews of their current and former employers, sharing insights around pay, benefits, and working conditions. When it comes to perceived ageism, a common complaint among workaday Americans, it can't all be gaslighting. Where there's smoke, there's ire.

In the acclaimed 2020 Shalini Kantayya documentary *Coded Bias*, MIT Media Lab researcher Joy Buolamwini investigates the bias in algorithms after uncovering flaws in facial recognition technology. It's chilling stuff: Technology doesn't see dark-skinned faces accurately. Admittedly, career recruiters and human resources departments use different types of algorithms to winnow through thousands of résumés and narrow the pool of candidates for a job. But it's all code, and if the code is biased or otherwise flawed, we've got a problem.

Imagine you're destined to live into your 100s; you feel the need to earn income in your seventies, eighties, or even nineties; and technology, along with the normal vagaries and challenges of age, is conspiring against you.

Paul Irving, a former president of the Milken Institute nonpartisan think tank and founding chair of its Center for the Future of Aging, predicts population aging will be the number two global concern after climate change. "The shifting demography will change everything," he says. And smart companies will grasp this: "The customer of the future is older. The employee of the future is older."

Irving, who is in his early seventies, sees two conflicting visions of our aging planet: One of sadness, chronic disease, dementia, loneliness, and isolation; and the other of hyperbole about living fulfilling 200-year lives or even living forever. "And I think the truth lies somewhere in the middle," he says.

"We're not just a society segregated by race and class—we're a society segregated by ageism," he says. It flows both ways: Not just millennials expressing "Okay boomer" contempt at their elders, but boomers who tell jokes about millennials and make disparaging comments about supposedly fragile Gen Zers.

At the United Nations, as world leaders take turns giving speeches that lay out what they see as the most pressing concerns confronting humanity, Bolivia's president spends part of his time at the podium decrying the lack of a universal treaty protecting older adults. But Luis Alberto Arce Catacora is an exception. Few other members of the world body broach aging at all, even though the UN High Commissioner for Human Rights has spoken out emphatically against the mistreatment of seniors who have been, in his words, "deprived of their liberty"—especially those confined to cramped quarters in nursing homes.

And in America, a nation where structural racism and ageism overlap, two worlds are colliding. Age bias isn't just buffeting the people who need nursing care—it's also affecting those who've been hired to feed them, bathe them, and empty their bedpans.

Robyn Stone, a former deputy assistant secretary for aging and long-term care policy at the US Department of Health and Human Services who is now a leading researcher at the University of Massachusetts Boston, says the millions of people who work as elder caregivers are chronically underpaid "because of an underlying sense of ageism."

"It's undervalued to work with older adults," she says. "They're going to get dementia. They're all going to die at the end. You can't get wages raised and compensation raised if nobody values the work."

Dr. Timothy Farrell, who chairs the American Geriatrics Society's ethics committee, agrees. "In this country we have a long history of racism, ageism, and an intersection of structural racism and ageism that impacts the quality of health care, including poor access and poor outcomes," he argues.

Researchers at the University of Michigan asked people aged fifty to sixty about their experiences with everyday ageism. Eight in ten respondents said they'd encountered one or more forms of it. Some also said they'd struggled with internalized ageism—thoughts like, "I'm older—I can't do that—that's for you younger people."

New York Times opinion columnist Pamela Paul captures this perfectly:

> It's all those little moments: waking up after a really good long night's sleep only to feel worse off than you did when you got into bed the night before. You don't bounce out but instead heave yourself up to audible snaps and crackles. You learn that you can inflict a grave injury to your own body simply by reaching for the alarm clock in the wrong way. You know that when you wind up in physical therapy it will not be the result of a marathon or water-skiing but because of something that happened on a sidewalk.

> Boomers, we know, didn't appreciate getting long in the tooth. They're the ones who started this whole fight against Old. But as a Gen Xer, I have to assume it's worse for us. Our entire gestalt is built around an aura of disaffected youth. There is no natural progression for that energy into middle age. I don't see us easing into words like "seasoned" or "mature." Millennials will no doubt take their own kind of

offense to aging when it's their turn, but that is not our cross to bear.

Even pop culture can't agree on whether longevity is a good thing. For every Bob Dylan ("Forever Young"), Oasis ("Live Forever"), or Pearl Jam ("Immortality"), there's a Queen ("Who Wants to Live Forever") or a Taylor Swift ("I Don't Wanna Live Forever").

In a rapidly aging world where more of us than ever before are going to have a legitimate shot at 100, we really need to get over purely artificial milestones like age sixty-five.

"Sixty-five is not old!" says Karon Phillips, a public health gerontologist with the Trust for America's Health. "We think of sixty-five as the retirement age, but that's not even the case anymore. Some people continue to work, or if they do retire, they go consult. Aging is not a monolith. We're not all aging in the same way."

ONE STRATEGY, ADMITTEDLY NOT ALL THAT ENTICING TO MANY OF us: If you're working now, don't stop.

She's an imperfect example, because she lived a life of immense privilege, but Britain's Queen Elizabeth II was ninety-six and had been sovereign for seventy years when she died in 2022. "One of her legacies is what it means to age, stay current, and remain relevant," says Gary Officer, president and CEO of the Center for Workforce Inclusion in Silver Spring, Maryland, which advocates for the needs of workers who are fifty and older. That's a sizable and growing bloc: In 2024, workers aged fifty to fifty-four represented the largest single segment of the American workforce.

There are compelling examples of ordinary folks who are still happily employed even though they've hit or surpassed 100.

A striking example is Ginny Oliver. At 104, the Maine native is still baiting traps and measuring and banding lobsters hauled from the frigid waters of Penobscot Bay—a job she started when she was an eight-year-old girl. The oldest licensed lobster trapper in the state, along with one of her sons—Max, the "baby" at age eighty-one—motors out three mornings a week in the *Virginia*, a boat that bears her name, to tend to her traps. "I've done it all my life, so I might as well keep doing it. . . . I'm going to retire when I die," she says.

Joe Smith is a kindred spirit. You might have expected that after fifty-seven years on the job at St. Clair Realty in Bakersfield, California, he'd have called it quits well before he became a centenarian. But you'd be wrong: When Smith turned 100, he shrugged off any thoughts of retirement. "I like to keep my mind busy," says the World War II Air Force veteran, who started working at age six on the family farm in Arkansas.

Perhaps no centenarian worker has challenged stubborn ageist sensibilities quite like Carmen Herrera, a Cuban-born abstract artist who died at her Manhattan apartment in 2022 at age 106. Herrera labored in obscurity for most of her life, finally gaining international fame at eighty-nine. "In an art world that worships the new and the young, Ms. Herrera advanced into old age ignored by the commercial markets, savoring only the solitary pleasures of all struggling artists: creating wonders for their own sake," the *New York Times* wrote in an obituary.

Dagny Carlsson, a Swede dubbed the world's oldest blogger, worked up until a few weeks before her death at 109. She wrote about her life based on a simple premise: Never think you're too old to do what you want to do. Carlsson launched her blog when she turned 100 and had thousands of followers. In her final post, in which she said she was looking forward to celebrating her 110th birthday, she flashed her sense of humor and lust for life: "Like a cat, I have at least nine lives."

And there's no shortage of celebrities coming up behind these remarkable "can't stop / won't stop" centenarians, suggesting we'll be inspired for decades to come. TV's borderline naughty, sometimes saucy Betty White led the way, and nearly until the end, *The Golden Girls* star was cracking us up. (Hilariously, she had the last laugh: When she died at ninety-nine, two weeks before becoming a centenarian, *People* magazine was already on the newsstands with a splashy but premature cover: "Betty White Turns 100!")

Beverley Johnson, one of the original supermodels, made history nearly fifty years ago when she became the first Black woman to grace the cover of *American Vogue*. Now seventy-two and a grandmother, she strutted the catwalk during New York Fashion Week in 2022,

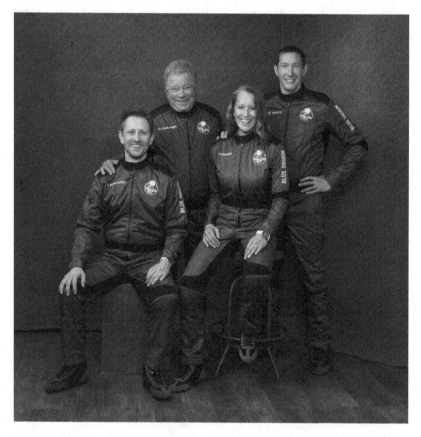

At ninety, *Star Trek* actor William Shatner was the oldest living person to travel into space for real. (*Blue Origin*)

displaying poise, class, elegance, and, yes, beauty. Cheering and clapping erupted.

Star Trek actor and author William Shatner is still creating at ninety-three. The man known to millions as Captain Kirk is discovering that age—not space—is the final frontier. Within a matter of months, he not only blasted off into space on one of Jeff Bezos's Blue Origin rockets, but he also released *Boldly Go*, a new book about that experience and his myriad others over T-minus nine decades and counting. ("So, I went to space," he deadpans, mock-flippantly, before waxing poetic: "I discovered that the beauty isn't out there; it's down here, with all of us.")

At ninety-two, legendary composer John Williams—the musical genius who's given us the themes to *Fiddler on the Roof, Jaws, Star Wars, Schindler's List,* and other blockbuster films—became the oldest-ever Oscar nominee for the score for Steven Spielberg's *The Fabelmans.*

A dozen years older than Williams, the dynamic nun known as Sister Jean inspired people on and off the court as the chaplain for the Loyola University Chicago men's basketball team that reached the NCAA Final Four in 2018. At 105, she released a bestselling memoir, *Wake Up with Purpose! What I've Learned in My First Hundred Years.*

And *Murder, She Wrote* star Angela Lansbury, who died five days shy of her ninety-seventh birthday, entertained us nearly all that time. Although she was often cast in older roles, the woman who sang the theme song for the animated movie *Beauty and the Beast* drew the line at playing "old, decrepit women." "I want women my age to be represented the way they are, which is vital, productive members of society."

What they've all had in common: a refusal to accept the ageist notion that once you hit your fifties, sixties, or older, you're all washed up. Angela Lansbury was a beauty, not a beast. But that's not the message our culture is sending to people her age.

• • • •

WANDER THE GREETING CARD AISLE AT YOUR LOCAL DRUGSTORE OR supermarket, and you'll see what I mean. It's open season on older people. Birthday cards declare us "over the hill" and depict us bent over and wrinkled, using canes or walkers.

When I turned fifty, a friend gave me a card that contained a miniature set of false teeth. Someone else gifted me a card concealing a tiny tube of hemorrhoid cream. Imagine if those crass gags poked fun instead at people's skin color, disability, or sexual orientation. Just think of the whirlwind we'd reap as a society.

Changing the Narrative, a nonprofit group campaigning to reframe attitudes around aging, has been calling on greeting card designers and others to ditch cheap-shot negative stereotypes that mock and marginalize older people as "sleepy, crabby, and weak," and instead celebrate them and their contributions, and the vital roles they play in society. "We need more messages that are clever and fun without all the age-bashing about sagging body parts and increasing irrelevance," it says.

It's not just the card industry. In 2018, the investment platform E*TRADE aired an incredibly tone-deaf and demeaning Super Bowl ad depicting eighty-five-year-old workers failing miserably at their jobs.

Martha Boudreau isn't laughing. As AARP's executive vice president and chief communications and marketing officer, she's on a mission to persuade society in general, and advertisers in particular, to stop using offensive and just plain inaccurate ageist tropes. Thirty-somethings are the creative directors at the vast majority of ad agencies, she says, yet few have ever been given a reliable readout on the fifty-plus demographic, let alone the sixty-plus or seventy-plus sets. That makes no sense, she argues, because it's those of us aged fifty and older who are powering the longevity economy. "Regardless of what you're selling, the fifty-plus are buying it," Boudreau says. "Why are marketers not understanding that?"

At least one company gets an AARP shout-out: Airbnb. The short-term rental giant has been airing a spot showing a couple in their seventies dancing and drinking champagne as they wander their romantic vacation villa, panning the next morning to the man in his pajamas, stretched out on the bed and sipping coffee. "It's wonderful!" Boudreau says. "It's just *wow*. Airbnb knows exactly who's renting that villa. They're looking at the data and they're seeing who they want to attract, based on who it is that's renting their properties."

Allure magazine, too, has gained admirers for trying to change the conversation by banning the term "antiaging" from its pages since 2017, even though it runs scores of skin care and beauty products pitched to women as ways to cosmetically turn back the clock. "Whether we know it or not, we're subtly reinforcing the message that aging is a condition we need to battle—think antianxiety meds, antivirus software, or antifungal spray," Michelle Lee, the magazine's former editor-in-chief, said at the time. "If there's one inevitability in life, it's that we're getting older. Every minute. Every second. . . . Yes, Americans put youth on a pedestal. But let's agree that appreciating the dewy rosiness of youth doesn't mean we become suddenly hideous as years go by."

AARP's Boudreau wants the advertising industry to use its enormous influence for good on aging in the same way its past campaigns helped reduce smoking and promote seat belt use. "Images matter. People see themselves or they don't," she says, applauding companies such as L'Oreal that feature brand ambassadors like eighty-seven-year-old Jane Fonda and seventy-six-year-old Maye Musk (yes, she's Elon's mother). "Their brand is elastic enough to be able to encompass a wider age segment with different products. It changes everything when you realize you're going to live half of your life over fifty."

And yet, somewhat awkwardly, even AARP acknowledges it doesn't put real people on the cover of its own magazine—not even those as remarkable as Sister Madonna Buder, a ninety-four-year-old nun who's the oldest woman ever—at age eighty-two—to finish an Ironman Triathlon. Why not? Because they're extreme examples and not, as Boudreau puts it, "aspirational within reach." Instead, the organization showcases celebrities, including stars who tend to be mostly on the younger end of its constituency: Adam Sandler, Viola Davis, George Clooney, Tyler Perry. "That's an age-old question: 'Why don't you put real people in the magazine?' Because the fact is, people don't want to see that. They want to pick up a magazine and go, 'Oh, wow,'" she says.

As a society, one way forward may be to combine young and old wherever and whenever possible. To do life together, intergenerationally, so boomers, Gen Zers, and everyone in between can experience the best the others have to offer.

Japan, so often an innovator in the aging space, is working to connect the very old with the very young. A nursing home in the city of Kitakyushu, in Fukuoka Prefecture, employs thirty-two "baby workers"—all of them under the age of four—who play, skip, and laugh in the presence of the facility's beaming older residents. Elders strike up conversations with the children, and vice versa; and the kids' parents or guardians are compensated with diapers, baby formula, and other gifts. "I don't get to see my grandkids very often, so the baby workers are a great treat," eighty-five-year-old nursing home resident Kyoko Nakano told the *New York Times*.

Perhaps it's a naïve wish, but it's difficult to imagine ageism continuing to take hold and fester if, like the organizers of the Japanese nursing home experiment, we become more intentional about creating spaces for mutual delight and appreciation across generations.

In Providence, which has a large and vibrant Latinx population, many families occupy all three floors of the city's numerous multifamily dwellings, and it's beautiful. Grandpa and grandma, *abuelo* and *abuela*, live on one floor, watching their kids' kids during the workday, knowing that when the time comes, their kids and their grandchildren will care for them. Three generations under one roof break bread and do life together. Maybe it's time for the rest of the country, including the wealthy white suburbs, to take a page from their playbook. It would certainly solve a lot of problems around elder care and aging in place—a happy ending most of us wish for, but that all too often becomes an elusive dream.

Some say it's a dream come true at Bridge Meadows, a privately and publicly funded multigenerational community on the outskirts of Portland, Oregon, which offers affordable housing to seniors, foster children, and their families. Derenda Schubert, Bridge Meadows' executive director, says the vibe is a village feel where families live intergenerationally in townhouses. It's her answer—really, more of a rebuke—to the United States having become a place where the generations no longer live or work in the same communities, much less do either of those things together.

"When you have people living adjacent to each other, and you have proximity and purpose, you're more likely to develop those really important relationships that become, over time, like family," Schubert says. "We are eliminating ageism because this child now sees this elder as someone I love and I want to take care of, and it's my duty to be involved with this person."

On a larger scale, though, the United States is no Japan—not even a Portland or a Providence—when it comes to sensibilities around aging.

"The United States is not a country known for valuing and honoring the elderly for their wisdom. It is more youth-oriented," the prominent American psychiatrist H. Steven Moffic writes in a commentary for the *Psychiatric Times*. "Countries where the elderly are valued, such as Japan, have what may be the world's longest life spans. . . . Over five centuries ago, the explorer Ponce de Leon was said to be trying to find the Fountain of Youth. Now we have finally found one of those fountains, but it is not a beverage, but a belief that bubbles over, a belief in the value of aging. Let's call it the 'Attitude of Youth.'"

Linda Fried, who directs the Robert N. Butler Columbia Aging Center at Columbia University, agrees. The United States, Fried says, is the most age-segregated society in the world—not a good thing when more of us than ever before will have a shot at celebrating our 100th birthdays.

"We've actually done the unimaginable and added thirty years to human life expectancy," and maybe even forty years, she says. "How do we grapple with the fact that we have a society that was not designed for longer lives? . . . We need each other across generations. We're all in this together."

WE BEGAN BY INVOKING JANE GOODALL, WHOSE BOUNDLESS ENERGY at ninety embodies what life can be in the ninth decade and beyond. Her inspiring and contagious sense of purpose recalls another tireless almost ninety-year-old: one who devoted the last three decades of her own life to fighting ageism, age discrimination, and other social ills swirling around older people.

At a time when no one would have faulted her for retreating quietly into obscurity and despair, Maggie Kuhn responded to her forced retirement at sixty-five from a job she loved at the United Presbyterian Office of Church and Society by starting a movement. Hell hath no fury like an activist scorned. Instead, Kuhn redirected her anger into founding the Gray Panthers, a loosely organized series of multigenerational, local advocacy networks. Since 1970, the Panthers have been confronting age bias and other social justice issues, and half a century later, they're still clawing away, changing the way the world looks at seniors. Kuhn died in 1995 at eighty-nine, exactly the age she'd hoped to make her exit. One of her most memorable quotes still resonates today: "Speak your mind even if your voice shakes."

It's not easy walking away from your lifework, but after considerable thought and some insightful conversations with family, friends, and colleagues, I've decided to make my exit while I can still do so on my own terms. It's women like Jane Goodall and Maggie Kuhn, and my own wife, son, and daughter, who've kindled within me an excitement to continue creating and contributing in a kinder, gentler, more reasonable rhythm of working. Toxic stress is the enemy of longevity, and the news industry is rife with it. I'll happily leave running a newsroom behind.

I'm not a mystic, but a poem by a fellow journalist is helping me make peace with this decision, and I'm enjoying the delicious irony of that. Peter Prengaman recites "Have You Done What You Wanted to Do?" in a kind of Eminem-esque rap cadence, and I'd be lying if I said it isn't speaking profoundly to me at this crossroads in my life:

Have you done what you wanted to do?
I ask because the time is upon you
It's upon me too
As human beings we have limited time
To do what we want to do
Close your eyes; seconds, minutes, and hours pass
The march of time is relentless, so fast
The present is all we have
But yet we bet on a future
It's a lure, a cure, to think
"I'll do this or that in the future for sure"
But will you? Or will your time be through
Before you do what you want to do

It goes on in this vein, and then he delivers this telepathic tercet
I just haven't been able to shake:

Inside you, you know what to pursue
Even if it would require a personal revolution
A self-made coup

IN MEDICINE, AS IN THE SOCIAL SCIENCES, MANY PHENOMENA TURN
out to be linked.

Experts call them the *social determinants of health*: economic stability; educational access and quality; health care access and quality; neighborhood and environment; and social relationships and
interactions. You don't just have a heart attack; you have it because
of your genes, your diet and exercise, and your stress levels. And all
those things depend on whether you're struggling to put food on the
table; can't afford to buy fresh, nutritious options; don't have time to
exercise because you're working two jobs; and worry so much about
paying your bills, the stress unleashes inflammation throughout
your body, damaging your heart and arteries over time.

Likewise, ageism isn't merely unjust, unhealthy, and immoral—
it's also a leading cause of loneliness.

Dr. Becca Levy, a Yale professor and a leading expert on the psychology of successful aging, argues that a solution for addressing
loneliness on the individual and structural levels is to reduce ageism.
Levy says we start forming negative stereotypes about older people
when we're as young as age four, and those stereotypes morph and
intensify as we age until we finally begin believing the distortions
and lies we've heard from others and ourselves. "We've found that
negative age stereotypes can lead to worse mental health, such as
depression" and even dementia, she says.

Some centenarians languish in loneliness and isolation. Others somehow navigate and overcome it. If we're destined to live to 100, is there anything tangible we can do while we're younger to position ourselves for camaraderie and connectedness?

Read on: The answers may surprise you.

CHAPTER SIX

SILVER WITHOUT THE LINING

The house I grew up in once pulsed with the happy chaos of life's daily dysfunction. Today, with my mother as its sole occupant, it's mostly quiet, save for the low-volume chatter of a TV that's almost always on somewhere.

There are three screens: one in the kitchen, another on the back porch, and a third in Mom's bedroom. My younger brother and I each drop in once or twice a week, but she's ninety-three now, so those TVs are her most faithful companions. Dad's been dead for more than two decades, and tragically, we lost our middle brother two years ago.

For Mom, who has buried both parents, a husband, a son, three siblings, several nieces and nephews, and too many friends and neighbors to count, longevity comes with a curse. It is the dull ache of loneliness—reflected in every framed family portrait; every personalized calendar; every faded, oxidized Polaroid snapshot taped to the side of the fridge. They're gone, and she's still here.

"See that TV right there? That's my companion. It keeps me company," she tells me, flipping over the playing cards laid out in rows on her kitchen table as she concludes a game of solitaire. Perched on the windowsill above the sink are two of her favorite coffee mugs.

One says: "What a Beautiful Day—Now Watch Some Bastard Louse It Up." The other imparts a singular truth she has so drummed into us for our entire lives, we've come to view it as a biblical imperative—a twenty-first-century *Thou Shalt Not* delivered via Moses straight from Sinai: "Jersey Girls Don't Pump Gas."

You'll recall her own mother lived very nearly to 104, and my mom—lean, spry, and active—seems to have inherited at least some of my grandmother's staying power. Joining the ranks of centenarians herself, though, is a thought she finds particularly off-putting. Our conversation about that begins like this:

"Mom, how do you feel about living to 100?"
"<unprintable>"

AS WE'VE SEEN, SOME SUPER-AGING RESEARCHERS THINK WE HAVE the potential to live to 150, although even if that's possible, it's likely a long way off.

Many in the scientific community understandably distance themselves from pronouncements by extreme aging provocateurs. I'm talking here about the likes of the English biomedical gerontologist Aubrey de Grey, whose theory of "Methuselarity" envisions a day—perhaps as soon as 2036—when medical technology will eliminate death from age-related causes. Or the American inventor and futurist Ray Kurzweil, who believes that if the human genome is basically a computer running outdated software, immortality is achievable by upgrading our operating systems through gene editing and other means. (Starting in 2029, the Google engineer predicts, medical advances will add a year—every year—to our life expectancy.)

It seems the mainstream scientific trend lines are shifting in those directions. In a 2021 study published in the peer-reviewed journal *Demographic Research*, Michael Pearce and Adrian Raftery of the University of Washington conclude it is "extremely unlikely" that a person will attain an age between 135 and 140 by the end of this century. But they also believe there's a strong likelihood that someone will live to between 125 and 132 years by 2100. Their research is powered by the International Database on Longevity created by the Max Planck Institute for Demographic Research in Rostock, Germany, which tracks supercentenarians in Canada, Japan, the United States, and ten European countries: Austria, Belgium, Denmark, England and Wales, Finland, France, Germany, Norway, Spain, and Sweden.

A separate team led by Timothy Pyrkov, a Singapore-based Russian scientist working with colleagues in the United Kingdom and the United States, also published work in 2021 suggesting a range in maximum human longevity somewhere between 120 and 150 years. And a study done the previous year by geneticists and others at Harvard Medical School and Moscow's Skolkovo Institute of Science and Technology produced an oddly specific maximum life span: 138 years.

What researchers don't discuss as much is whether 150 is worth the effort.

No one in recorded history has ever lived that long. Imagine outliving even your oldest loved ones by up to half a century. Even those who've hit 100 say the pitfalls can easily outweigh the benefits: debilitating medical conditions, a loss of independence, and the loneliness that comes with vastly outliving spouses, children, and friends. Eventually, as significantly more of us age into triple digits, we'll have more company. But a society where 100 is the norm is decades away—and until then, many centenarians will have to reckon with some measure of solitude.

"I've been forgotten by our good Lord," France's Jeanne Calment ruefully said as she approached 122, having painfully outlasted those closest to her. A devout Catholic, the woman some geriatricians nicknamed "the Michael Jordan of aging" often spent her mornings in prayer, asking God a simple, plaintive question—one we'll never know whether He answered:

Pourquoi? Why?

Across the Atlantic, most Americans sixty-five and older say they'd happily live to 100 and beyond, but only under certain conditions, and more than half worry that old age is too risky to be worth the trouble. A Harris Poll of 2,022 US adults found that one in nine people sixty-five and older would like to reach 100 only if they could be certain they'd have a sound body and mind. Eight in ten say they'd like to become centenarians if their spouses or partners were still alive. And lest we think vanity fades with age, seven in ten of us say we'd be fine with 100, so long as we'll wind up looking younger than our age. But, and here's the catch, 59 percent of us think there are just too many unknowns to make living that long worth it.

Part of the problem, two University College London academics argue, is how we frame extreme aging. "Very old age, if commented upon, is presented as if it were a kind of extreme sports competition," Paul Higgs, a professor of the sociology of aging, and Chris Gilleard, a visiting research fellow in psychiatry, write in an essay for *The Conversation* about the darker side of living to 100. "Centenarians are celebrated simply for reaching 100. Nonagenarians hit the news when they run a mile, climb a mountain, or pilot a plane. Otherwise, silence reigns. . . . The social networks of the frail elderly, whether living at home or in a nursing home, tend to be so much smaller than those of the rest of the population. Most people over eighty live alone. They often have only a few people to talk with. Aged lives of quiet desperation are sadly not rare."

All the lonely people. The Beatles were certainly on to something with "Eleanor Rigby."

Life extension, still mostly theoretical, muddies the equation. Historically, the rich are in a far more privileged position than the rest of us to take advantage of anything and everything that lengthens life, whether it's cryogenics, experimental treatments, or the 3D bioprinting of replacement body parts. Need a heart, a liver, a lung, or a kidney? Forget about transplantation lists and donor shortages—just have your doctor right-click and send that job to the printer. It's quickly moving from science fiction to fact: In 2022, a twenty-year-old Mexican woman born with an undersized and misshapen right ear underwent successful surgery to attach a 3D living tissue copy of her left ear. It was printed in ten minutes by bioengineers at 3DBio Therapeutics, a regenerative medicine company in Queens, New York, using a collagen-based "bio ink" containing some of the patient's own cells to ensure the replacement ear regenerates cartilage. How much would an implant like that cost when such procedures become more commonplace? Notably, the company won't say, leaving us to guess about the future availability to the masses of 3D-printed vital organs when those eventually become viable.

Polls consistently capture deep-seated skepticism over whether such life-extending breakthroughs will be within reach of anyone who isn't wealthy. An overwhelming number of respondents to a Pew Research Center poll expressed their belief that everyone should be able to get life-extending treatments, but two in three said they think only the rich, in practice, would have access.

John K. Davis, a professor of philosophy at California State University, Fullerton, has written extensively about the ethics of life extension. He posits this not-so-hypothetical question: Imagine you have wealthy neighbors who can afford expensive life-extending measures and will live to 190. You can't, and you're dying at eighty when you'd hoped to make it at least to ninety. Is your death not so bad, for you're losing only a few years, or is your death now far worse, because—if only you had life extension like the rich folks next door—you might live to 190? Are you losing ten years or are you losing 110 years?

A record number of Americans say they've gone without health care over the past year because they couldn't afford it—yet the wealthy are spending millions on supposedly rejuvenating stem cell treatments. "In a world where money can buy almost everything, going to elaborate lengths to extend life itself while so many Americans suffer without health care might just be the ultimate form of conspicuous consumption," writes *Washington Post* columnist Helaine Olen.

Others in the scientific community stake out even more blunt positions. "Research with the explicit aim of extending the human life span is both undesirable and morally unacceptable," concludes Martien Pijnenburg, a medical ethicist at Radboud University in Nijmegen, the Netherlands. His principal beef: How can anyone justify extending the lives of wealthy Westerners when billions in the developing world already perish prematurely in what's become known as unequal death?

And in an otherwise dry academic treatise on the pros and cons of artificially gaming the system to gain a few more years, Pijnenburg poignantly pivots to the very essence of the loneliness question: "Human beings cannot live without meaningful relations with others. Goods that are essential for a good life, such as friendship, are essentially goods that are bound to the social dimensions of life."

Sociologists Iliya Gutin and Robert A. Hummer of the University of North Carolina at Chapel Hill echo that, cautioning against unjust efforts to extend life expectancy "in a high-income but enormously unequal society like the United States, where social factors determine who is most able to maximize their biological life span." Translation: If a longevity dystopia awaits us, we'll likely find ourselves stuck between two unsavory extremes—elitist checkbook life extension and populist "eat the [old] rich" outrage.

Reflecting on his career at age eighty-three, as he lay dying of cancer, the late *Boston Globe* reporter and columnist Jack Thomas recalled one of his most memorable stories, one about a centenarian who'd outlasted her children. "I interviewed a sweet woman, 101 years old, who was annoyed at God, and she intended to give him a piece of her mind. Her greatest grief was not her pending death, but the fact that she had outlived her four sons. 'I can't imagine what God had against me that he would take them before me,' she said. From the mantel of her fireplace, with trembling hand, she lifted a photograph of each son and kissed it."

Underscoring how much we need one another—and how that interdependence affects our physical and emotional well-being—US Surgeon General Vivek Murthy has proclaimed loneliness a global public health crisis. One in three older adults feels lonely, the World Health Organization confirms. And all that solitude is taking a toll on our minds and bodies that experts liken to the deadly effects of obesity or alcoholism. The National Institute on Aging says the health risks of prolonged isolation are equivalent to smoking fifteen cigarettes a day and may shorten a person's life span by as much as fifteen years. Like stress, it can trigger inflammation throughout the body and elevated levels of cortisol and other hormones that can increase blood pressure.

"Loneliness acts as a fertilizer for other diseases," Steve Cole, director of UCLA's Social Genomics Core Laboratory, tells the NIA. "The biology of loneliness can accelerate the buildup of plaque in arteries, help cancer cells grow and spread, and promote inflammation in the brain leading to Alzheimer's disease. Loneliness promotes several different types of wear and tear on the body."

Loneliness, by the way, isn't the same thing as being alone. Introverts like me can attest to the restorative power of withdrawing from others to recharge. When I need a break from the rest of you, I go for a long run, a solo day sail on Narragansett Bay, or steal away for some fly fishing where it's just me and the trout—all solitary pursuits. But those are personal choices. Loneliness is the inner anguish that springs from craving companionship and camaraderie only to be deprived of them. Researchers have found evidence of a greater likelihood of depression, suicide, dementia, Alzheimer's disease, a compromised immune system, and a heightened incidence of heart attack and stroke among seniors who complain of feeling lonely. They're also more likely to develop low self-esteem and feelings of guilt or worthlessness. And extroverts in general, multiple studies have shown, tend to outlive introverts—great news for my wife, a social butterfly; for me, not so much.

"You can certainly be alone without feeling lonely," says Janine Simmons, a psychiatrist and neuroscientist at the National Institute on Aging. But aloneness is on a continuum, and like pretty much everything else extreme in life, excessive solitude depletes us. It's why some societies, and many Americans, view the solitary confinement employed at US prisons as cruel and unusual punishment; and why elders confined to their homes with little or no human contact can feel similarly imprisoned. "We need connections with other people to survive and thrive," Simmons says.

"Lacking social connections can increase your risk for premature mortality from all causes," adds Julianne Holt-Lunstad, a professor of psychology and neuroscience at Brigham Young University and an expert on loneliness and social isolation.

Okay, fine. But centenarians, by definition, already have defied death. For them, it's more a quality-of-life question. Even if they've only got a few more years, they're no less interested in life, liberty, and the pursuit of happiness. To be sure, given what they're up against physically, mentally, and emotionally, those things can be elusive.

At her 120th birthday party, Madame Calment stoically told reporters: "I see badly, I hear badly, I can't feel anything, but everything's fine." She'd pedaled her bicycle around Arles until she turned 100, and lived on her own until she was 110, only to spend her last seven years confined to a wheelchair; her famously long mobility and independence forever behind her.

Researchers at Cambridge University in the United Kingdom were curious about centenarians' psychological well-being, so they studied ninety-seven people ranging in age from 100 to 108 to see what role anxiety played in their daily lives—specifically, if they were experiencing enough anxiety to make it "clinically relevant" to their overall health. Nearly half had anxiety at clinically significant levels, resulting in a worsened perception of their own health, a higher number of medical conditions, financial worries about the cost of treatment, and loneliness. "Feeling lonely may predispose centenarians to (develop) clinically significant anxiety and be important to their overall well-being," the researchers concluded.

A much larger study of older adults in Amsterdam found that social loneliness was significantly associated with a reduced chance in women of reaching the age of ninety. Men didn't seem to be affected quite as much, possibly because women are more likely to be widowed and to wind up living alone. "This indicates that, for women, a large and diverse personal network at an older age could increase the probability of reaching longevity," the researchers conclude, though they say more study is needed.

Our default way of thinking about life is that more is better. How could it not be, we ask ourselves. Consider John Keats, the great English Romantic poet, who didn't live to see his twenty-sixth birthday; or the Renaissance painter Raphael, who died on his thirty-seventh. Surely their brief life spans deprived us all of even more beauty. Even so, considering the drawbacks and downfalls of vastly outlasting our contemporaries, is it really worth it?

It's complicated, says Dr. Lisbeth Nielsen, director of behavioral and social research at the National Institute on Aging. Nearly 14 million older Americans live alone, yet many of them are neither lonely nor socially isolated, Nielsen says. Scientists are still figuring out how loneliness affects health, and why so many centenarians somehow navigate and overcome it on their way to achieving exceptional ages.

"Centenarians are vulnerable and resilient at the same time," concludes a team of researchers at Fordham University who've studied the effects of loneliness and social isolation on centenarians and near-centenarians. A New Zealand study, meanwhile, finds that centenarians are 32 percent less likely to feel lonely than people in younger elderly groups, such as those sixty-five-plus—perhaps because of the mental toughness and coping skills they've acquired through having endured more of life's difficulties.

And there's a subset of seniors who haven't been unwillingly isolated by society. It's a lifestyle, for better or worse, that they've chosen and embraced for themselves.

My mother is a bit like this. We've asked her countless times to consider moving in with us. My wife and I even bought our current home with her in mind—it's got a spacious ground-floor bedroom and an adjacent walk-in shower—but she won't have it. She's content to live independently in the home she raised her kids in, for as long as she can. Mom's refusal to let us look after her exposes an irreconcilable generational divide you'll find in most American families: Many in my generation, the boomers, are more than willing to take in our aging parents and spare them the indignities of a nursing home; and many in hers, the Silent Generation (generally defined as people born between 1928 and 1945), would rather die than feel like they're a burden to their children.

Social media can provide a measure of connection, as flimsy and superficial as it is. But for people of a certain age, like my mother, it's a mystery they've never bothered to figure out. It's still difficult to imagine even for me as her son, but in her ninety-three years, she's never owned a computer or a smartphone, or sent or received a single email, let alone friended or followed anyone or "liked" anything online. Her house is wired for cable but not Wi-Fi. Some days I'm aghast; other days, I'm envious. She has, after all, been entirely spared the vagaries of being sucked into the soulless social media vortex with its attendant mindlessness and misinformation. Unlike her, today's tech natives—tomorrow's nonagenarians—will experience their nineties and beyond in fully wired fashion.

In the 2015 Academy Award–nominated film *A Man Called Ove*, based on the novel of the same name by Fredrik Backman (and just remade by Sony Pictures as *A Man Called Otto* starring Tom Hanks), the title character is an isolated curmudgeon who spends his days visiting his wife's grave and hating on pretty much everyone else. "Whatever we do in this life, no one gets out of it alive," he grumbles. Fortunately for Ove, a young family who moves in next door and won't take no for an answer persists in making contact until he lets them in, literally and figuratively.

Not that seniors are the only ones combating loneliness. Millennials and Gen Zers were suffering in silence even before the COVID-19 pandemic, which took everyone's social isolation to a new low. Research shows people aged eighteen to twenty-four are at a high risk of loneliness and also least likely to take action: a dangerous combination.

At least two nations—Britain and Japan—are responding to loneliness whenever and wherever it may be found by making it a major government priority. Both countries have created a cabinet-level "Ministry of Loneliness" to address isolation across all population groups. Within Japan, meanwhile, the conversation has taken on a macabre tone: So many seniors are dying alone—their remains sometimes not discovered until weeks or months later, requiring elaborate and expensive fumigation of their apartments—that landlords are demanding elderly tenants use wearable devices that can transmit their vital signs and other information to agencies that monitor their well-being.

In the United Kingdom, "we're still in a critical stage when it comes to tackling loneliness," says Baroness Diana Barran, who served as her country's first loneliness minister, implying that, collectively, we may reach a more comfortable spot on the societal solitude scale when many more of us are older.

The British effort has focused heavily on TikTok and on catchy hashtags like #LetsTalkLoneliness on other social platforms—not exactly places where centenarians and other exceptionally old individuals typically congregate. But at least it publicly acknowledges the loneliness that multiple generations have suffered in darkness and silence. In a clear indication of their sincerity and determination to tackle the issue and erase the stigma around it, both the United Kingdom and Japan—demographically one of the world's oldest societies—have committed to meet regularly and learn from each other. Barran and her Japanese counterpart, ex-minister Tetsushi Sakamoto, see loneliness as an important international challenge, and connecting family, friends, and neighbors as a vital step in overcoming it.

Calls for a similar approach are coming from other countries, including South Korea, which has one of the highest suicide rates among developed nations. "There is a growing demand that Korea as a society needs to address the issue of loneliness," says Noh Woong-rae, a Democratic Party of Korea lawmaker.

Eddy Elmer—a Dutch Canadian gerontologist whose research has found that loneliness "causes a wear and tear on the body that becomes more pronounced over time"—cautions that even efforts intentionally targeting seniors often fall short, if only because key segments of the older population are missed. "In trying to foster social connection, much of our focus has been on the 'low-hanging fruit,' like people at senior centers," says Elmer, who's based in Vancouver, British Columbia. "We overlook those who want to be socially connected but are homebound, introverted, or don't consider themselves seniors. Cities must increasingly focus on reaching older adults where they are."

In progressive and innovative Vancouver, where my son and his wife live and work, officials have been experimenting with "naturally occurring retirement communities"—sizable communities of seniors who decide to age in place rather than move into retirement homes. For those who find themselves isolated in high-rises, Vancouver has a "Hey, Neighbor" program that pays a stipend to apartment dwellers who are willing to serve as social concierges, helping coordinate transportation and home services for seniors and connecting them to outings and social events in the building. "We can give incentives to developers to incorporate sociable design in new buildings, such as common rooms, outdoor seating, and intersecting pathways. And postal carriers, police, and firefighters might start getting to know people in their neighborhoods through community events," says Elmer, a board member of the British Columbia Psychogeriatric Association. "In an era of fiscal deficits, these initiatives may seem like luxuries, but for those with no social contact, they can be lifesaving."

From the earliest days of human civilization, we've been trying to fix this loneliness problem. Perhaps no one personifies this more than poor Job, the Old Testament figure who loses his children, his wealth, his health, and very nearly his mind:

> I go about in gloom, without any sunshine; I stand up in public and plead for help.
> My voice is as sad and lonely as the cries of a jackal or an ostrich.

Jeanne Calment was born in 1875, the year Leo Tolstoy published his first installments of *Anna Karenina*, considered by many to be the greatest novel of all time. After the title character commits adultery, she's snubbed by polite society and languishes in social isolation:

> How they looked at me, as at something dreadful, incomprehensible, and strange! . . .
>
> There was no answer, except the general answer life gives to all the most complex and insoluble questions. That answer is: One must live for the needs of the day; in other words, become oblivious.

THE UNKNOWNS, AND POTENTIAL DOWNSIDES, OF LIVING TO 100 and beyond make my mother an unwilling centenarian in the making.

She was born in 1931 in Paterson, New Jersey, to parents of sturdy Sicilian stock. My grandfather, Joseph Sansone, emigrated from Sicily as a young man and served with the Army in World War I. Later, he worked as a grocer, housepainter, and Christmas tree salesman. I was only seven when he died at sixty-seven, but I still remember Grampa Joe's ebullient laughter and the way he'd spontaneously break into song. It's my Brooklyn-born grandmother, though, who had the star power—and the longevity. As a young woman, Concetta Marie Mercurio was a pianist for silent movies and an accomplished toe dancer who performed onstage in New York City. She'd eventually outlive her husband by nearly four decades; something her Sicilian parents never could have imagined. And now her daughter, Marie "Nadine" Kole, is making her own uneasy way along the road to 100.

"I don't feel like my age. I feel much younger than my age. I feel maybe sixty," she tells me, flashing some annoyance when I mention she's in her early nineties. "I still do my own stuff. I still go shopping. I do my own errands, and I drive to the supermarket."

This makes me very nervous. When my mother turned ninety-one, her driver's license expired, so she went to the Registry of Motor Vehicles in Massachusetts to renew it. I expected them to give her a road test to reassess her skills. Secretly, I hoped for it. But no—they simply gave her the usual vision check, and after she demonstrated no need for corrective lenses, they issued a new license that won't expire for *five years*. She'll be ninety-six then. Will they renew it again so she can legally drive when she's 101? How can this be sound public policy?

Statistically, although drivers aged eighty or older get into fewer wrecks overall, they're involved in the most traffic fatalities per mile traveled. Only two states, Illinois and New Hampshire, require those aged seventy-five and up to take a road test when they renew their licenses. The rest rely on a loose system of "self-selection"—counting on older drivers to give up driving on their own when they're no longer confident of their physical strength, cognitive abilities, or reaction times. Frankly, that seems dubious, especially for older seniors in rural or suburban areas where public transit is limited or nonexistent. A few years ago, my mother voluntarily stopped driving at night and on highways, and she confines her trips to a roughly five-mile radius of her home, all of which, it must be said, is thickly settled. But expecting her to surrender the keys entirely? That's unrealistic in a country where mobility and independence are inextricably intertwined. As we all barrel collectively toward 100-year life spans, elder driving is an issue we need to address at the state and national level.

I have a vivid memory of my grandmother when she was about my mother's age—in her early nineties—and we were all on the dance floor at my brother's wedding. There, to our astonishment, she kicked her feet up to the height of our shoulders, busting moves I couldn't do in my thirties. "What an unbelievable lady," Mom tells me. "She

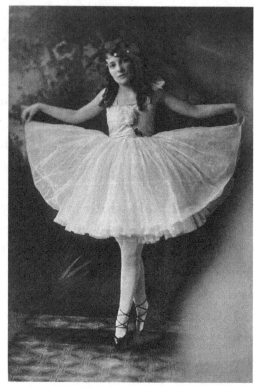

Marie Sansone, the
author's grandmother,
circa 1920.
She was born in 1899 and
died in 2003, just shy of
her 104th birthday.
(*Author family photo*)

was a wonderful person. I think anybody would want to take after her, honestly."

But she's ambivalent about living to 103: "I don't think about living so long. I just enjoy my life. When your time is up, it's up. That's it."

When will her time be up? I ask.

"How do I know? I don't know."

When will *my* time be up?

"Oh God, I hope not for a long time. . . . We never know those things. Maybe it's better not to."

Drilling deeper into her misgivings about achieving centenarian status, it's the loneliness factor that gives her most pause.

That makes sense, says Anne Basting, the founder of TimeSlips, an international network of artists and caregivers who are committed to bringing more joy and meaning to people in the twilight of their lives. She's part of a growing movement of organizations that are investing time and resources into older people regardless of their perceived value to the economy. When human beings of any age cease contributing to overall economic productivity and lose the focus of capitalism's lens, she says, we don't know how to value them. That's when we start viewing them through the crass and narrow lens of the medical system, rather than as people with extraordinary knowledge and experience—gifted souls who can volunteer, mentor, and lift others to new heights.

"The big issue is avoiding isolation," says Basting. The United States, she notes, is particularly bad at providing seniors with transportation and leveraging our current systems—everything from postal services to meal delivery, telephone wellness checks, and even voting—to create what she calls "meaning-making" and connectivity for our oldest citizens. "We are," she says, "a species that's hungry for meaning."

"Simply say, 'hello,' and remember it's the little things that can make a difference" in the lives of older adults who live alone, says Sandra Harris, who cochairs the Massachusetts Taskforce to End Loneliness & Build Community. "We know how important it is to connect." In that same spirit of doing little things to foster connection, the city of Salem, Massachusetts—borrowing an inexpensive but effective strategy that's succeeded in the United Kingdom—has set up a dozen "Happy to Chat" benches in public parks. It's a designation that lets lonely seniors and others know the stranger sitting on that particular bench is open to conversation.

Some countries, notably Japan—where, as we've seen, nearly a third of the population is sixty-five or older—are using artificial intelligence glibly known as "agetech" to help their elders stay mentally engaged. The architects of Japan's system call it Society 5.0, and they see robotics and AI as answers to the dual challenges of a rapidly aging society and a dwindling labor force. The Japanese government articulates its vision to become "a super-aging and supersmart society" by integrating technology into elder care. Increasingly, because of a chronic shortage of caregivers, sensors are monitoring the well-being of seniors in nursing facilities as well as those aging in place in their own homes. AI even initiates a phone call to a doctor or a social worker if the sensors warn that something's off.

But is AI a realistic and practical substitute for actual human touch, empathy, tears, laughter, and the milk of human kindness? Basting isn't so sure. "[Meaning-making] can be assisted by AI, but it has to have a human component to it somewhere," she tells me. "When you create an architecture around these systems for meaning-making and loneliness, that meaningfulness has to come in somewhere." And Basting raises more existential questions that all the futuristic, gee-whiz-holy-shit technology in the world will never be able to answer.

"The big challenge when you get to the nineties and the 100s is the 'why,'" she says. "Why have I been given these final years? How do I use them? Is it enough just to watch TV, or engage with the AI companion, or the robotic seal, or the baby doll? What is the 'why'? Loneliness is different at different parts of your life. There can be a sense of, 'God has forgotten me, all my friends are dead, all my family is gone.' Some people outlive even all their own children. That kind of loneliness is a different thing, and we have to understand it with a different lens."

If it's any comfort to those of us destined to outlast our loved ones, they're never truly gone—not as long as we carry them within us. Whether we'll draw sufficient solace at 100 from our memories of those who may have predeceased us will, of course, depend on us.

Even the great Elisabeth Kübler-Ross, the Swiss American psychiatrist and author whose pioneering study of loss gave us the five stages of grief—denial, anger, bargaining, depression, and acceptance—claimed in the latter part of her life to have connected spiritually with long-dead loved ones. At the end, she even, in a sense, disavowed the acceptance stage of grieving, because she found that her dear ones were, at some mystical level, still with her. Here's Basting, channeling Kübler-Ross: "They're still there with you. They're meaningful to you. Just be with them and talk to them. If people are present in your memory, that's a really interesting thing."

One virtue of aging in place—something we'll explore in greater detail in chapter 9—is that under the right circumstances, loneliness doesn't even have to be part of the extreme longevity equation. In many immigrant enclaves, communities of color, and other pockets of our population, multigenerational homes are the norm: Elders live in close proximity to their children and grandchildren, who not only provide care but conversation. It can be, and often is, a beautiful and elegant solution for all parties involved, not just the elderly.

At Bridge Meadows, generations step up in turn to help one another. "It's grandparents raising grandchildren," director Schubert says. Then the roles reverse: The community's children check up on and care for its older residents. "When you have people living adjacent to each other, and you have proximity and purpose, you're more likely to develop those really important relationships that become, over time, like family," she says. "It's about creating a safety net of neighbors supporting neighbors. We're taking care of each other."

That, in fact, may be part of the secret behind the blue zones we'll examine more closely in the last chapter of this book—those handful of places that, for reasons not entirely understood, seem to produce substantially older, substantially healthier seniors. The only US blue zone, you'll recall from chapter 3, is Loma Linda, California, a center of the Seventh-day Adventist Church, whose members tend to live a decade longer than other Americans. Tom Perls, our longevity expert at the New England Centenarian Study, notes that its adherents model a number of healthy habits. Most are vegetarians or vegans; they don't drink or smoke; and their weekly sabbath is truly a day of rest. But the shared trait that interests him most is that they interact with one another constantly in extended social groups. "They tend to spend quite a bit of time with family and religion, which may help them manage their stress better than others," he says.

AS WE AGE, OUR EMOTIONAL RESILIENCE—THAT ENIGMATIC X FACtor that's helped Holocaust survivors go on to reclaim their lives, and those who've overcome earthquakes or even physical and emotional abuse to rebuild theirs—is something we can tap to handle whatever challenges a 100-year life may throw at us.

Dr. Laura Carstensen, director of the Stanford Center on Longevity, led a study that examined the well-being of older people during the COVID-19 pandemic. The scourge, of course, exacted a terrible toll among the elderly—far and away its most frequent and numerous victims. "We found that older people reported fewer negative emotions in their lives, and more positive emotions, than younger people did," Carstensen tells NPR's *On Point*. "It isn't the fact that there aren't older people who are struggling emotionally, but there are many fewer of them struggling emotionally than young people." It's even more nuanced than that: "Older people have more mixed emotions. They're more likely to experience joy with a tear in the eye than younger people are. We see a kind of a savoring and an appreciation—that's what captures the emotional experience. It is not a uniform, simplistic happy." Carstensen elaborates:

Older people are affected by terrible things, just as younger people are. But they come to that with experience, and they come to that with a perspective. And if I may say just a word about both, the experience that comes with age allows us to know that bad times pass. There's a sense when something negative happens that you've been here before, and that this time will pass. There's another change that occurs with age and that's that we become increasingly aware of our own fragility. We become aware of our own mortality as friends and loved ones die, as we recognize that life doesn't go on forever. And if there's a paradox of aging, it's that when we recognize the limitations on life, rather than become anxious and depressed, we savor them. We know that bad times pass and we know that good times do, too. And so, the good times are savored. . . . And we have a kind of a strength that is difficult to achieve in a very short life. We have a strength of social connections and experience that allows us to brace during very, very difficult times.

Perls, too, has found centenarians to be inspiringly positive. Most of those who live to 100 or longer tend to have a good handle on stress, and they're agreeable and optimistic. (Much more on the relationship between positivity and extreme longevity in the last chapter.)

There's one segment of the population that's especially susceptible to loneliness, and it's both growing and aging: LGBTQ+ seniors.

Older Americans who identify as nonbinary, especially those living in rural areas, are discriminated against in multiple ways, says the National Resource Center on LGBTQ+ Aging, the only organization of its kind in the United States that focuses specifically on improving the quality of services and support offered to lesbian, gay, bisexual, transgender, or queer older adults, their families, and their caregivers. In 2010, the center says, there were an estimated 3 million nonbinary seniors in the United States; by 2030, their numbers are projected to grow to 7 million—more than double. Britain, too, is dealing with a rapidly expanding LGBTQ+ community that's also disproportionately affected by loneliness. Officials there say Britons who identify as gay or lesbian are one and a half times more likely to be lonely, and those who identify as bisexual are two and a half times more likely.

The isolation can be brutal, and many are unlikely to have access to health care and social services that are openly inclusive of LGBTQ+ older adults. "It leaves many LGBT older adults feeling like they must hide who they are in order to take advantage of health and social service programs," says Sherrill Wayland, the National Resource Center's director of special initiatives. "Many are not comfortable about letting others know about their sexual orientation or gender identity." Being nonbinary in a city doesn't always help: One in four gay, lesbian, bisexual, or trans seniors in New York City say they have no one to call in case of an emergency.

In a powerful essay for the *Washington Post*, Steven Petrow describes how, for many LGBTQ+ seniors, the latter years are far more fraught than golden.

"We're twice as likely as our straight counterparts to be single and live alone, which means more likely to be isolated and lonely. We're four times less likely to have children. We're more likely to face poverty and homelessness, and to have poor physical and mental health. Many of us report delaying or avoiding necessary medical care because we face discrimination or mistreatment by health care providers. If you're queer and trans or a person of color, these disparities are heightened further," he writes.

Imani Woody, a longtime advocate for women, people of color, and the LGBTQ+ community, is building Mary's House for Older Adults in her childhood home. The not-for-profit organization in Washington, DC, creates welcoming and inclusive environments for LGBTQ+ elders and helps them deal with social isolation and loneliness in part through community living. "It's hard to be old and gay," says Woody, who's been honored with AARP's Purpose Prize. Some same-gender-loving seniors, she cautions, "are going back into closets of despair, fearful and isolated. It's just sad."

"I know the difficulties that come with aging as a gay person, because I *am* a gay person, and I *am* aging," she adds.

For gay and straight elders alike, aging also often includes hearing loss, and that accentuates an affected individual's sense of isolation and loneliness. "As you get older, your chance of having age-related hearing loss is almost certain," says Dr. Justin Golub, an ear, nose, and throat specialist and age-related hearing loss researcher at Columbia University. And yet it's rarely treated or covered by health insurance—something Golub finds "incredibly puzzling."

Sufferers "withdraw from society. . . . They sit in their room and stare at the ceiling." He quotes Helen Keller, who said: "Blindness separates us from things, but deafness separates us from people." One bright spot: US health regulators' recent rule allowing Americans to buy hearing aids without a prescription—a long-awaited move intended to make the devices more accessible to millions with hearing problems.

WHAT IF, AS WE'VE EXPLORED, THERE'S NO EXPIRATION DATE ON human existence? Would it make our lives better or just longer?

Mackenzie Graham, a research fellow in philosophy at the University of Oxford, suggests we'll need to weigh the pleasure of extra time against the pain: "There could be many circumstances in which we might live for too long. Sometimes it might be better for us to die earlier than we otherwise might have, if doing so is more consistent with the life story we wanted for ourselves—for example, being active and independent throughout our lives."

Graham's observations take me back to the early 1990s, when I was a journalist based in Detroit and wrote extensively about the late Dr. Jack Kevorkian, his suicide machine, and the spirited national conversation around individual end-of-life decisions. Kevorkian, a

retired pathologist, helped about 130 ailing people—many suffering from chronic and debilitating pain—end their lives. American
society wasn't ready to accept the idea of physician-assisted suicide
even in such desperate cases, and Kevorkian, demonized by some
as "Dr. Death," was imprisoned for eight years. Today, he's widely
credited with helping nudge hospice care into the medical mainstream. I'll never forget sitting in his lawyer's office and watching
grainy videotape of two feeble, disabled women who desperately
wanted to die and did so in a secluded Michigan cabin using devices
Kevorkian invented. Amid tears and laughter, they recommitted
to their decisions on the eve of their deaths. One of the women said
something so raw and searing, I can't help but recall it whenever I
hear a conservative pastor or talk-radio pundit smugly rail against
the supposed immorality of euthanasia: "I tried loading a gun, but I
didn't know how to load one. If you do it yourself, you don't know what
you're doing." Another thing I'll never shake is something Kevorkian
himself once said about the taboo obscuring the notion of death with
dignity: "Dying is not a crime."

Must aching loneliness, sharp physical decline, and a painful
and protracted death dominate our living-to-100 highlight reels?
Not necessarily.

As the entire population continues to age, all boats rise, leaving
open the possibility of this tantalizing (and, let's face it, appreciably
more cheerful) alternative reality: We may find ourselves growing
exceptionally old in the company of our contemporaries. And if that
happens, it changes everything.

Especially, as we'll explore in the next chapter, as our bodies *and*
our minds withstand the ravages of extreme aging.

CHAPTER SEVEN

TRIPLE-DIGIT BODIES; DOUBLE-DIGIT MINDS

Every Tuesday, like clockwork, I used to get an invitation from Jesus Christ.

It was the late 1990s; I was the Associated Press bureau chief for the Netherlands; and one of our now-obsolete office fax machines would shudder to life before producing a single sheet of ink-streaked paper that instantly curled into a tube like a Dead Sea Scroll. It always read the same, in crisp, formal Dutch: Jesus would be holding his weekly press conference in The Hague at 11:00 a.m. He would be discussing current events and the end of the world, and he would be taking questions. I was cordially invited.

I never went, and more than once, I've joked that I dearly hope I won't end up regretting that decision. People always laugh, as they do when I recount the accomplished older ex-journalist I knew in Holland who, in the dimming twilight of her life, went from bar to bar dressed in a ball gown and loudly introduced herself as the Queen of England. Or the eccentric Bostonian who emailed me weekly for a year, insisting that federal agents had rented the apartment below his and were feeding fiber-optic cable through their ceiling—his floor—to keep him under surveillance.

I chuckle, too. Over the years, like many journalists, I've stuffed hundreds of anecdotes like these into an ever-thickening "weird shit" file. At one point, I'd even considered writing a book about the most unusual of my encounters with self-styled celestial prophets and other unconventional characters. The working title: *JOURNALOONYISM.*

Truth be told, though, it's not funny. There's nothing amusing about mental illness or delusions, especially those that manifest in old age. All too often, the fog of memory loss, confusion, and disorientation can give way to full-blown dementia, sometimes with startling personality changes. It's the cruelest of jokes: miserable for patients robbed of their very selves, heartbreaking for families, and an absolute nightmare for caregivers.

Florian Zeller's moving 2020 Academy Award—winning film, *The Father,* holds up a mirror to the tensions and turbulence of navigating that world. In a poignant performance that won him an Academy Award for Best Actor, octogenarian Anthony Hopkins captures the bewilderment of a real-life descent into dementia, complete with conversations with imagined individuals as the fabric of reality frays:

> [Sobbing] I want my mommy. I want my mommy. I want to get out of here. I want her to come and fetch me. I want to go home. . . .
>
> I feel as if I'm losing all my leaves. . . . The branches and the wind and the rain. I don't know what's happening anymore. Do you know what's happening?

My own grandmother was spared the worst of that on her slow march nearly to 104, but there's something my family seldom talks about: Toward the end of her majestically long life, she no longer knew who my mother was.

At least she managed to dodge dementia's onset for a decade and a half longer than statistics suggest most of us can expect. The average age for people in the United States to begin experiencing symptoms is 83.7. Doctors say those who develop dementia also are at greater risk of other serious health problems such as diabetes and a heightened risk of stroke.

Yet as we find ourselves propelled into a new era of exceptional longevity, there's increasing hope that some—perhaps many—of us will experience the gold standard of super-aging: reaching 100 with reasonable physical fitness and the mental sharpness of someone half that age, with no significant signs of dementia.

REMEMBER 113-YEAR-OLD HERLDA SENHOUSE, WHOM WE MET IN chapter 4? She's already made arrangements to donate her brain to be studied after her death. Based on the lively conversation she and I had in her apartment about food, faith, and politics, researchers will find none of the plaques and tangles that are the calling cards for Alzheimer's and other brain-wasting diseases. Or, if they do, they'll discover she escaped the effects unscathed.

She's living proof that mental decline and dementia don't have to be part of the extreme longevity equation. Researchers call centenarians and supercentenarians like Herlda "cognitive super-agers," and although her astonishing age makes her exceptional, a surprising number of people 100 and older share her mental acuity.

What do these people do to both grow so old and stay so sharp? Among other things, it turns out a majority of those who attain exceptional ages demonstrate extraordinary resilience in the face of stress, says Emily Rogalski, a super-aging expert at Northwestern University's Feinberg School of Medicine, who for a decade has been

studying people aged eighty through the 100s. "The super-agers'
brains look indistinguishable from a group of healthy fifty- to
sixty-year-olds. They really seem to be on a different trajectory,"
Rogalski says. Her latest work is evaluating super-agers' life stories
to get a better idea of how they've handled stress, whether it has
involved surviving a Nazi death camp, coping with the death of a
child, or dealing with cancer. She's noticed a theme emerge: "We all
encounter stress and have the opportunity to react in different ways.
One reaction can be to rise above, and it seems like these super-agers
are particularly good at identifying the best in a situation and figuring out how to move on."

Adding an element of wonder to whatever cognitive super-agers
have going on, they're doing it despite the tangible changes that occur
in our brains as we age.

A ninety-year-old's brain typically weighs 1,100 to 1,200 grams—
nearly 10 percent less than a forty-year-old's brain. That shrinkage
we experience later in life primarily affects the prefrontal cortex and hippocampus as well as the cerebral cortex, a part of the
brain used for complex thoughts. But people who attain exceptional
ages have been found to have a thicker cingulate cortex, a region
believed to play an important role in attention, cognitive control,
decision-making, and memory. Super-agers' cerebrums also have
been shown to include many more corkscrew-shaped *von Economo*
neurons, which are involved in rapid communication across the
brain, and their brains just generally seem to handle the wear and
tear of aging better. What's still not entirely clear: Are centenarians
born with larger, stronger brains? Or are they somehow able to acti-
vate a response to aging that compensates for the brain degradation
others experience over time?

A new study of 340 healthy Dutch centenarians living independently finds they "experienced no decline in major cognitive
measures, except for a slight loss in memory function" akin to what

one might expect if they were in their seventies. Some of the studied centenarians, in fact, had brains that appeared very healthy, and they performed at a high level on cognitive tests. Others who died with no discernible degradation of their memories or their abilities to relate to others and solve problems had their brains examined, and here's where it gets wild: Their gray matter was as marred and scarred as that seen in people who die with advanced Alzheimer's, yet their brain function was never compromised. And the oldest of these folks was 108.

"Some individuals reach ages beyond 100 years and become centenarians with intact cognitive functions, which indicates that cognitive impairment is not inevitable at extreme ages," concludes the team at Vrije University in Amsterdam led by Dr. Henne Holstege. How is that even possible? They're not sure. "It is still unclear to what extent individuals who maintain cognitive health until age 100 escape or delay decline," the researchers say, adding that 40 percent of us will develop dementia by the time we turn 100. If that sounds bleak, you can take comfort in this: 60 percent of us won't.

Once we're 100, though, the risk gets markedly higher. A person who lives between 100 and 102 has the same chance of acquiring dementia as a person living between seventy and ninety-five. Put another way: Twenty-five years of risk in that slightly younger population, Holstege's team says, is compressed into two years in centenarians. It also means that centenarians who never develop dementia should be considered that much more extraordinary.

And new work by an international team of researchers who scanned data collected from 101,457 brains ranging from a 16-week-old fetus to a 100-year-old is revealing that the brain adjusts as we age to help us meet the challenges of every stage of our lives.

"For those who are cognitively intact at about 100 or 101, they really seem stable for a significant period of time," says Tom Perls, who's been closely tracking the Dutch project. "It's as if they've demonstrated their ability to be resilient against a disease or even resistant against it. At that point, they just keep on going. They plateau. It's only when we start to see a decline in their cognitive function that we start to get worried."

Perls says the Dutch experience points up these realities about extreme old age: Debilitating brain disease is nowhere near as inevitable as it once seemed, and many super-agers appear to be resistant, resilient, or both.

It's good news that loss of cognitive function as we age isn't guaranteed, considering memory loss, Alzheimer's disease, and dementia affect more than 50 million people globally and another 12 to 18 percent of people sixty and older live with mild cognitive impairment. Nearly 10 million new cases are diagnosed every year, though a new study from the RAND Corporation says the prevalence of all types of dementia dropped by nearly a third in people older than sixty-five from 2000 to 2016. In the United States alone, more than 6.2 million people are currently coping with Alzheimer's—a national caseload the federal Centers for Disease Control and Prevention expects to more than double by 2060. But it's not hitting equally: Over the next forty years, Latinos are projected to see the steepest increase in cases. One recent study warns that America's Latinx population can expect a sevenfold greater prevalence of Alzheimer's by 2060—a trend researchers believe may be linked to the high incidence of diabetes and high blood pressure among some Latinos. (Another study offers a silver lining: Many US Latinos are bilingual, and there's evidence to suggest speaking a second language builds "cognitive reserve" that may help the brain bear up better under Alzheimer's.)

Alzheimer's, the most common cause of dementia and the fifth leading cause of death in adults older than sixty-five, slowly destroys memory and thinking skills. Eventually, the fatal neurodegenerative disease robs sufferers of the ability to carry out the simplest of tasks. Noticeably more women than men are diagnosed with it;

the recent discovery of a gene that appears to put them at greater risk may explain why two-thirds of the Americans currently battling Alzheimer's are female. New research in Australia that examined data from eleven countries involving nearly 4,500 people aged ninety-five-plus suggests women globally are especially vulnerable. People who've been infected with COVID-19 also appear to be at a substantially heightened risk—82 percent higher for women and 50 percent higher for men.

And the costs of care are enormous: an estimated $305 billion in the United States in 2020. As the population ages, that's expected to triple to more than $1 trillion.

This grim backdrop is what's motivating Perls and Boston University behavioral neuroscientist Stacy Andersen to figure out why some centenarian men and women are as cognitively alert and intact as their peers who are thirty years younger, and why Alzheimer's hasn't impacted them. One day, they say, it could lead to a vaccine against the disease or a pill to treat it.

"Not all centenarians have dementia and, perhaps even more significant, about one quarter of the population has no cognitive impairment" at all, Andersen notes in a 2020 study that investigated them as models of resistance. "A centenarian who is cognitively healthy at age 100 has a high probability of remaining cognitively healthy until death."

In fact, supercentenarians—the elusive 110 and older set—spend on average only 5 percent of their entire lives dealing with an age-related disease. By studying 500 high-functioning centenarians, Perls, Andersen, and George Murphy, codirector of the Center for Regenerative Medicine in Boston, are working to unlock how people aged 100 and older remain intact.

"Despite the fact that aging is one of the strongest risk factors for cognitive impairment, aging in centenarians is typified by resilience and in some cases resistance to age-related disability," Perls says.

"We aim to discover genetic variants and biological mechanisms that protect against aging-related brain changes and Alzheimer's, and then translate those findings into therapeutic strategies and targets."

A separate and ambitious new study led jointly by Perls, the Albert Einstein College of Medicine in New York, and the American Federation for Aging Research is enrolling 10,000 people aged ninety-five and older in a quest to learn more about the role of genetics in aging slowly, living longer, and keeping debilitating diseases like Alzheimer's at bay. That study will compare traits in super-agers and their children to traits in older adults whose parents did not achieve exceptional ages, and, also important, it will create the world's largest single biorepository database for future research into healthy aging. "We're just now getting up to speed. The next few years are going to produce a tremendous amount of clinical and biological data," Perls tells me.

Such super-agers are, as we've discussed, "black swans"—exceptional beings who, by rights, ought not to exist but nonetheless do.

"For most of human history, centenarians were a rare and unpredictable phenomenon," say a group of Italian geriatricians examining the growing population of people in their 100s who somehow manage to remain mentally sharp and physically active. Healthy centenarians, they say, "are a living example of successful aging free from chronic diseases causing permanent injuries and from reduced mental and physical functions."

"Generally, they reach 100 years of age in good health, and only after 105 years of age start to manifest age-dependent alterations," reports that team, based at the University of Catania. And it notes something else: Supercentenarians have a lower incidence of dementia than "younger" centenarians. Almost as an afterthought, the team warns of "enormous social, economic, and health impacts" as millions age into triple digits with the considerable staying power of robust health. Society, it cautions, needs to undertake "a drastic revision of education, health, employment, retirement, and other policies," if we want a better sense of the global impacts.

Centenarians are also surprising us with their physical stamina. It's something to think about the next time you're tempted to help that little old lady or gentleman cross the street.

Virginia McLaurin, who died recently at age 113, epitomizes the extraordinary things centenarians are capable of. She was 107 when she burst onto the national scene after dancing with the Obamas during a visit to the White House. Video of their impromptu encounter went viral; a good thing, since she'd barely been making ends meet. Her newfound fame prompted strangers to donate enough to a crowdfunding campaign for her to move to a better apartment and get new teeth and a new wig.

At 105, Earl Mallinger was one of America's oldest farmers. His secret to a long and healthy life is straight out of Herlda Senhouse's playbook: Don't stop moving. Not long before his death, Mallinger still tended to the sugar beets, wheat, and soybeans on his thousand-acre farm in Oslo, Minnesota. Others handled the field work, but he still called the shots. "Keep moving. Once you quit moving, you'll go downhill pretty fast," said Mallinger, who had more than sixty grandchildren and great-grandchildren. His other advice: "Don't sweat the small stuff."

These centenarians amaze, inspire, and confound us. They exemplify what's coming: exceptionally long, exceptionally full, exceptionally astonishing lives.

But let's be real: Few of us, me included, see ourselves waltzing or farming or running marathons in our 100s. Trust me when I say I'll probably feel no need to run 26.2 miles as a centenarian, though I'd certainly love it if I could step outside now and then to get a little fresh air and walk 0.2. I'm pretty sure I'd be more than content to live independently and in reasonable health, able to move with relative ease around my home and neighborhood, so long as I could still interact emotionally, intellectually, spiritually—in a word, *fully*—with the people in my life.

That's what makes the latest research so encouraging. Finally, there's some real hope that new drugs in development may slow the progression of Alzheimer's. And new blood tests could change the way we approach diagnosis and treatment.

But what's the difference between loss of memory due to ordinary aging and the onset of dementia or Alzheimer's? It's a question I've been asking myself as I keep close tabs on my mother.

AT DAWN ON A RECENT AUTUMN MORNING, AFTER OVERNIGHTING AT my mom's house, I lace up my running shoes and put in six quick miles before showering, downing a quick cup of coffee, and rushing to the train station to catch the 7:53 to Boston. As I head out the door, I wish her a great day.

At lunchtime, my iPhone rings. It's Mom, and she sounds anxious. "Billy? Are you okay? You never came back from your run, so I'm just checking to see where you are." In the space of a few hours, she's forgotten we had coffee and I'd left hours ago for the office.

Many of us have had interactions like that with our older loved ones. Is it dementia? An early sign of Alzheimer's? Or just mild forgetfulness, on par with losing track of our car keys? The Alzheimer's Society's frustrating but accurate answer: It depends. Patterns offer much more insight than any single incident or behavior.

For instance, it's normal to occasionally forget an appointment, an acquaintance's name, or a friend's phone number and recall the information a short time later. Someone living with dementia, however, may forget things more often, or have difficulty recalling information they've recently learned. It's one thing to leave the house on a wintry day without a hat or gloves; it's another entirely to stand frozen in front of the mirror, suddenly unsure of how to get dressed. Anyone, from time to time, can struggle to find the right word to express what they want to say; someone with dementia may forget simple, everyday words and substitute others in a way that can make it difficult to understand them. All of us have momentarily forgotten what day of the week it is, or why we went into a room; that's different from getting lost on our own street, with no idea how we got where we are or how to find our way home.

There are many more such distinctions. Not seeing a doctor right away if we don't feel well is understandable; failing to get immediate medical attention if we're bleeding profusely or suffering chest pain could be a deadly mistake. Balancing a checkbook can briefly confuse anyone; forgetting what numbers are, and what they're used for, is a warning sign that something more profound is amiss. Who hasn't misplaced a purse or a wallet? That's benign; stashing your wristwatch in the coffee tin or your clothes iron in the freezer isn't. Ditto sudden and inexplicable mood swings, or personality changes that are out of character, like when a loved one with a typically sunny disposition becomes confused, suspicious, or withdrawn. Most of us, from time to time, temporarily get sick of tidying up the house or following through on social obligations; someone living with dementia may "check out" for much longer periods of time and need to be coaxed into reengaging with others.

There's no ambiguity for those who care for a demented loved one. They know exactly what they're dealing with, and it can be gut-wrenching.

Patti Greco, a writer I know, captures that powerfully in "This Is Our Long Goodbye," an evocative blog post about grieving all that she and her father have lost in his years-long descent into dementia:

Grieving the loss of a person with dementia is like death by a thousand cuts. You watch your loved one vanish a little bit at a time—sometimes in ways that are perceptible only to you, other times in ways even a stranger would notice—and you never know when another piece is going to break off. It just does, and you have to accept it and adjust your care plan, or deny it and suffer the consequences.

Mentally running my mother through the Alzheimer's Society's helpful checklist, I realize she's mostly exhibiting the kinds of momentary lapses that are typical of many people in their nineties. That's reassuring, and a neurological assessment by her doctor is even more so: She can readily recall the basic details of major life events, even as her short-term memory slips. And in a stroke of genius, my wife suggests an elegant solution for that: Now we jot down for her where we've gone on a yellow Post-it note as a reminder. So far, it's been working wonders, although Mom can find it exasperating at times.

"Take a pill," she tells me.

Ironically, one may finally be within reach—for you and me, anyway, if not for her.

CAN THE DEVASTATING PROGRESSION OF ALZHEIMER'S DISEASE BE halted, or at least slowed? An experimental new drug is raising hopes, though one of the labs involved has dashed that dream before.

In 2021, the US Food & Drug Administration ignored the objections of dozens of prominent scientists and fast-tracked its approval of biotech behemoth Biogen's much-hyped Alzheimer's drug, aducanumab. The FDA inexplicably cleared the drug, known commercially as Aduhelm, despite no conclusive evidence it slows the decline of memory or brain function in dementia patients. That touched off an internal furor: Aaron Kesselheim, a highly respected Harvard Medical School researcher, resigned in protest from an FDA advisory committee over what he called "probably the worst drug approval decision in recent US history."

A little over a year later, Biogen regrouped, partnering with Japanese pharmaceutical giant Eisai on another drug, lecanemab. A major clinical trial of the antibody treatment involving nearly 2,000 people with early Alzheimer's suggests a "clinically meaningful" impact on their brain cognition and function. There's a setback: Two participants in lecanemab's human trials have died. And a catch: Early versions involve getting a twice-monthly dose intravenously under a doctor's supervision, something that's obviously much more complicated than popping a pill or a capsule. But in the highly incremental world of Alzheimer's research, as in most scientific pursuits, even small advances are celebrated. In mid-2023, the FDA approved lecanemab, also known as Leqembi, citing evidence that it modestly slows the disease's early stages. What's far less clear: Who can afford

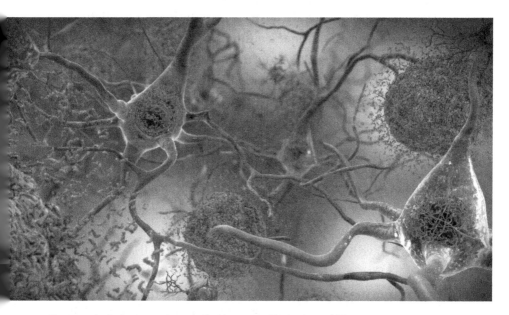

Beta-amyloid plaques and tau in the brain are telltale signs of Alzheimer's disease. (*National Institutes of Health*)

the estimated $26,500-a-year price tag, and how much of that will Medicare and private insurers cover?

During two decades of study involving billions of dollars, the focus has been mostly on amyloid plaques, which are believed to play a major role in the disease. Amyloid-beta is a naturally occurring protein, but in a brain afflicted by Alzheimer's, it clumps together to form plaques and tangles that researchers think disrupt communication among our billions of neurons. The same protein also appears to play a role in Down syndrome, and scientists say there's growing evidence that people with Down syndrome are at a higher risk of developing Alzheimer's as they age. (They're living longer, too: Life expectancy for a person born with Down syndrome in the United States was just twenty-five in 1983; today, it's sixty.)

In many scientific circles, though, you can color the experts decidedly skeptical. Biogen's failed Aduhelm, which, like lecanemab, targeted amyloid buildup, understandably has given scientists pause, and not only because it didn't live up to all the hype. Scientists have identified other Alzheimer's culprits besides amyloid, such as microglia, immune cells unique to the brain; a mutation in a gene called TREM2 has been found to weaken microglia and increase the risk of Alzheimer's. They're also rethinking the role that inflammation plays when it becomes too strong or doesn't go away. Given all that, a consensus is emerging that it will likely take a combination of medications—not just a single wonder drug—to defeat the disease. That's not stopping attempts: Researchers are experimenting with injecting a protective gene into patients' brains, so far with promising though inconclusive results.

There have been other disappointments as well: Late in 2022, the Roche Group subsidiary Genentech announced discouraging results from its trials of gantenerumab, yet another anti-amyloid drug. So far, the best we've managed to do—barely; *maybe*—is to slow the cognitive decline of Alzheimer's, not cure the disease outright.

On that front, there's more potential good news, and from an unexpected source: Researchers say natural compounds found in beer hops, which contain antioxidant properties, may provide a degree of protection. Hops, a University of Milan team finds, unleash "bioactive" molecules that go after amyloid-beta proteins and target some of the other early biochemical brain events that precede Alzheimer's development. If it turns out hops really *do* help protect against Alzheimer's, it will confirm a truth immortalized in one of my favorite quotations (never mind that it's routinely misattributed to founding father and avowed wine guy Benjamin Franklin): "Beer is proof that God loves us and wants us to be happy."

There are also early signs that eating or drinking foods that contain antioxidant flavonols—think beans, broccoli, kale, spinach, and tea—might slow the decline in memory as we age.

As the quest for a cure continues, others are investigating the roles exercise and brain training might play in reducing the risk of developing dementia.

Large-scale studies have shown that running, cycling, walking briskly, dancing, and other kinds of vigorous movement are keys to lowering dementia risk. Even something as humdrum as vacuuming your apartment or other household chores that get you moving can offer a benefit, new research suggests. One eleven-year study, which analyzed the health records of more than 500,000 Britons who did not have dementia, found that those who worked out or played sports were 35 percent less likely to develop it. Less active subjects who reported regularly attacking household chores had a 21 percent lower risk. The takeaway: If you spend three hours a week vacuuming, sweeping, and scrubbing strenuously enough to work up a sweat, you're very likely getting much of the same brain benefit as someone who devotes the same time circling the track or pumping iron at the gym.

Laura D. Baker, a professor of gerontology and geriatric medicine at Wake Forest University in North Carolina, studied 300 older adults with mild cognitive impairment—a condition she describes as a sort of "gray zone" between normal cognitive function and dementia. For a year, some were assigned high-intensity movement such as aerobic exercise; others did low-intensity activities that involved stretching and balance. "What we found was that neither group declined. This was a shock to us," she says. "Regular supervised exercise can protect against decline."

Baker ran another study in which 2,000 people were given either a multivitamin or a placebo daily for three years; those who got the vitamin showed measurably improved cognition, though more study is needed to confirm the connection. And her team has found something else: Prioritizing a good night's sleep, reducing sugar intake, refraining from smoking, drinking alcohol in moderation or not at all, and staying socially connected to others also appear to help preserve healthy brain function in older adults. (Don't overlook that sleep piece. A good night's rest appears to play a key role in living to 100. More than half of the centenarians in one study reported sleeping eight hours or more a night, and researchers have established a link between sleep duration and diminished accumulation of harmful brain amyloid.)

But what about those of us who can't engage in meaningful physical exercise—a situation just about everyone eventually will confront, depending on how deep into our 100s we end up living?

Scientists are trying to figure out if "brain training"—putting ourselves through video game–style thought exercises—can forestall or even prevent the onset of dementia. A first-of-its-kind US trial known as the POINTER study (the acronym is a confusing jumble of letters borrowed from Protect Brain Health Through Lifestyle Intervention to Reduce Risk) is enrolling 2,000 people ages sixty to seventy-nine nationwide to use software designed to test and strengthen participants' focus, attention, thinking reflexes, and memory. Organizers say it's an attempt to expand on findings from a recent study in Finland that reports a combination of physical activity, nutritional guidance, brain training, and social activities protected healthy older adults at increased risk of cognitive decline.

One of my questions, as I watch my mother read the newspaper and play solitaire, is whether certain kinds of brain training are more effective than others in slowing cognitive decline. Unfortunately, the answers are proving elusive. Many seniors and some clinicians swear by crosswords and other problem-solving puzzles like the *New York Times'* daily Wordle challenge, but past studies have yielded mixed evidence. One that followed several hundred nursing home residents in the Bronx, New York, found the crossword enthusiasts among them delayed the onset of accelerated memory decline by an average of two and a half years. Another that took a similar approach with people in late middle age living independently in Scotland didn't see a difference.

But a landmark study published in 2017—the first to show that any type of intervention, physical or behavioral, could lower the risk of dementia—found that healthy older adults who underwent a specific type of brain training known as "speed of processing" were nearly 30 percent less likely to develop dementia after ten years than people in a control group who didn't get the training. The training repeatedly exposes older adults to pictures presented briefly on a computer screen, and it's designed to enhance the speed and accuracy of their response.

Education appears to play a role in when, or whether, a person begins to experience mental decline. Researchers have found that people with college degrees are less likely to develop Alzheimer's and other neurodegenerative conditions, and there is evidence to suggest that continuing education—even studies pursued very late in life—offers some protection. Learning new information and skills throughout our lives, they say, is one way to lengthen them.

Elly Pollan, a long-retired accountant and great-grandmother from New York City, needs no convincing: At ninety-two, she earned a humanities degree from Lasell University in suburban Boston. "I wanted to continue my education. It's wonderful, actually. It keeps you alive and keeps you interested," she tells the *Boston Globe*.

For those who do develop dementia, artificial intelligence and machine learning are increasingly used to keep them cognitively engaged, and a new generation of smartphone apps is helping to guide them through daily tasks. One of these, MapHabit, uses visual mapping and audio prompts to walk dementia patients through simple but essential activities like showering, brushing their teeth, and taking their meds, then provides feedback to caregivers. The National Institute on Aging gave MapHabit's creators a shout-out and a $250,000 award for designing it to tap a relatively durable region of the brain that governs habitual memory rather than the hippocampus, which runs short-term memory and typically takes a hit very early in Alzheimer's. Another, Lumosity, offers fifty games and activities intended to improve memory, attention, and problem-solving. Millions have downloaded it and similar apps over the past few years, grasping hold of a digital lifeline that will become exponentially more commonplace as technology gives us new ways to grow older with dignity.

Meanwhile, if you find yourself anguishing over whether you or someone you love has Alzheimer's, simple new blood tests are now on the market that can confirm what you're up against. The tests detect minute amounts of amyloid and other suspect proteins in the blood. A few caveats: They're expensive; they're usually not covered by insurance; and if you or your loved one tests positive, there's not a whole lot you can do about it until medicine gives us effective treatments.

And, one day, a cure.

Please, God, I find myself praying, *let that eventual cure be permanent.* I've been haunted by scenarios in which regression follows progression ever since fourth-grade English class, when we read Daniel Keyes's heartbreaking Hugo Award–winning short story, *Flowers for Algernon,* about a developmentally disabled man who becomes a genius—temporarily—after undergoing experimental surgery:

> Just leave me alone. I'm not myself.
> I'm falling apart, and I don't want you here.

Thor actor Chris Hemsworth is among those who've subjected themselves to a more elaborate battery of genetic tests designed to gauge an individual's risk of neurodegenerative disease. Hemsworth's results show he carries two copies—one from his mother, another from his father—of the gene APOE4, which has been linked to an increased risk of Alzheimer's. Only 2 to 3 percent of the population have two copies, a kind of unenviable genetic double jeopardy where Alzheimer's is concerned. Hemsworth, who decided to be tested as part of *Limitless,* his new Netflix docuseries exploring the upsides of longevity, tells *Vanity Fair:* "There was an intensity to navigating it. Most of us, we like to avoid speaking about death in the hope that we'll somehow avoid it. We all have this belief that we'll figure it out. Then to all of a sudden be told some big indicators are actually pointing to this as the route that is going to happen, the reality of it sinks in. Your own mortality."

It's as though Hemsworth, in real life, is channeling his character in 2017's box office blockbuster *Thor: Ragnarok:*

> I choose to run toward my problems and not away.
> Because that's what heroes do.

· · ·

THERE'S A LOT AT STAKE FOR EVERYONE IN MINIMIZING THE INCI-
dence of neurodegenerative disease, and that's especially true for
those of us who hope to continue contributing meaningfully to
society in our 100s.

Delaying or avoiding mental decline is everything. Just ask Dr.
Howard Tucker—at 102, the world's oldest practicing physician.
Shortly after his 100th birthday, he became infected with COVID-19
at the hospital in Cleveland, Ohio, where he still puts in long days,
and continued to teach his neurology residents via Zoom. "I truly love
what I do," says Tucker, who began his medical career in 1947, when
Harry Truman was president. "The challenge of thinking through a
case and getting to help patients, as well as teaching the next generation of neurologists, never gets old."

Sure, but *he's* getting old. That prompted another physician, cardiologist Sandeep Jauhar, to ask a pointed question in a provocative
essay for the *New York Times*: "How Would You Feel About a 100-Year-
Old Doctor?" Nearly one in three American doctors is sixty or older,
and many have no intention of retiring. Jauhar doesn't advocate a
mandatory retirement age for doctors once they turn sixty-five or
seventy or some other predetermined age. But he does see merit
in the idea of requiring them to undergo a competency and skills
assessment that, just in case, could include screening for low-level
cognitive impairment. "It's important to be frank about aging,"
Jauhar writes, adding: "Age may be just a number, but it is one highly
correlated with physical and mental decline." (The centenarian doc's
cheery rebuttal: "After seventy-five years, I still enjoy contact with
patients. . . . Sometimes, patients request a second opinion. I tell
residents they shouldn't be disturbed if a patient asks, 'May I see an
older physician with more experience?' Eventually, they will hear
patients ask, 'May I see someone a little younger who knows all the
latest information?'")

Live long enough, however, and anything is possible. That's a principle we'll all be counting on as the years pile up and 100 draws nearer.

Renowned Dutch neuropathologist Wilfred den Dunnen has experienced that for himself. When he conducted an extensive assessment of 112-year-old Hendrikje van Andel-Schipper, not only was she free of symptoms associated with cognitive impairment, but she performed on par with a healthy sixty- to seventy-five-year-old. Den Dunnen found her to be "an alert and assertive lady, full of interest in the world around her, including national and international politics." Immediately after Ms. van Andel-Schipper's death at 115 years and 62 days, the world's oldest person at the time, den Dunnen carried out an exhaustive pathological examination of her body.

She'd contacted the University of Groningen when she was eighty-two to make sure her remains were donated to science, and when she turned 111, she phoned them anew to ask if they'd still have a use for such an old specimen. Absolutely, the researchers responded, trying not to sound too excited. They found she had virtually no buildup of plaque in her arteries and no Alzheimer-esque tangles in her brain. In death, as in life, she impressed: At 112, she had neurons in abundance, in numbers you'd find in healthy people aged sixty to eighty.

"Are there limits to the duration of high quality of life? Are there limits to healthy life for a human brain?" den Dunnen asks rhetorically.

None that were evident in Ms. van Andel-Schipper's case. Her improbably long life got off to a precarious start: She weighed a mere three pounds (1.36 kilograms) when she was born on June 29, 1890, half a century before modern neonatal intensive care units gave preemies a fighting chance. Yet she survived and thrived. As a little girl in 1898, she celebrated the coronation of Dutch Queen Wilhelmina; more than a century later, when she officially became the Netherlands' oldest living person, she found herself a guest of honor in the court of Queen Beatrix, Wilhelmina's granddaughter.

A die-hard soccer fan who rooted for Ajax Amsterdam, this spunky woman known to family and friends simply as Aunt Henny had her share of hardship: She had to sell all her jewelry to buy food during Germany's World War II occupation, and her husband died in 1959, leaving her childless and alone. Undaunted, she made a living teaching needlepoint, and lived on her own until she was 106, crediting her longevity to the daily consumption of a herring and a glass of orange juice (I suspect not at the same time). Nine years later, she was still happy and healthy.

She died peacefully in her sleep, the way we'd all like to go.

Cause of death: old age and a stomach tumor she didn't even know she had.

LET'S ASSUME FOR A MOMENT THAT YOU'LL REACH 83.7 COGNITIVELY intact, or already have. What are your hopes and dreams for however many years you've got left? It's something Americans have been collectively debating as well, with people taking sides on this provocative and not at all hypothetical question: Is serving as president of the United States a reasonable expectation for someone that age?

Octogenarian president Joe Biden's accelerated aging over the past couple of years alarmed millions of Americans, including many Democrats, who think eighty-something is just too old for the White House.

To those openly questioning Biden's vigor and mental sharpness, the president long responded with a two-word rejoinder: "Watch me." There are, however, considerations that go well beyond competence.

The average American's age is 38.5, and many key leaders are more than twice that age.

Few appear interested in taking a cue from Shakespeare's King Lear, who professed his intent

To shake all cares and business from our age
Conferring them on younger strengths, while we
Unburden'd crawl toward death.

Think of centenarians, and "feeble" often comes to mind. But our eldest elders have formidable political power—and it's only going to grow.

CHAPTER EIGHT

EXCEPTIONALLY OLD, WITH EXTREME INFLUENCE

Joseph Robinette Biden Jr. was 78.1 when he took the oath of office as America's oldest chief executive. Fun fact: My own modest and mercifully short-lived political career made history, too, but in my case, it was because of my youth.

In the mid-1970s, at the tender age of sixteen, I became the youngest town official in Foxborough, Massachusetts, with an appointment to the Stadium Advisory Committee. They couldn't have found someone less suited to civic affairs than the long-haired, clog-wearing, pot-smoking high school junior they brought aboard. But as a musician, I possessed vast knowledge of a niche my grumpy, bushy-browed elders on the committee readily conceded they were clueless about: rock 'n' roll.

The committee's job was to advise police, firefighters, and paramedics on what sort of crowds they could expect at Schaefer Stadium, the brutalist forerunner to today's gleaming Gillette Stadium, as the stadium owners warily began branching out beyond New England

Patriots home games to host concerts. My task, as the panel's only member fluent in contemporary music culture, was to offer informed opinions about such weighty matters of state as: Are Fleetwood Mac fans likely to ignore the Port-a-Potties and pee in the townsfolks' bushes? How rowdy are Jimmy Buffett buffs? What about those teeming hordes of tie-dyed Grateful Dead groupies—they won't *all* be smoking reefer, will they? (I had a hard time answering that one with a straight face.)

I'm the first to admit I didn't dazzle as a public servant. I wasn't exactly a young JFK. In fact, it's probably a good thing for my quaint little hometown that whatever oratory I may have delivered to urge expanded stadium beer sales went unheeded. Yet the town fathers' deliberate decision to slot my youthful voice into local government discourse—readily acknowledging they didn't know what they didn't know—was an elegant solution and an early experiment in intergenerational boutique politics.

As society ages in profound ways, we risk morphing into a full-blown gerontocracy that's indifferent to younger generations' needs, dreams, and desires.

In the United States of Graymerica, we're arguably already there.

THE UNITED STATES HAS HAD FORTY-SIX PRESIDENTS OVER ITS nearly two-and-a-half-century history. Their median age: fifty-five. The youngest POTUS to be sworn in was Theodore Roosevelt, six weeks shy of turning forty-three. The second-oldest: Biden's predecessor, Donald Trump, whose term began when he was seventy-and-a-half.

Depending on your own age and outlook, that's either inspiring or depressing. Either way, you'd best get used to it: Older Americans' lock on higher office is only going to intensify as the baby boomers age into their 100s.

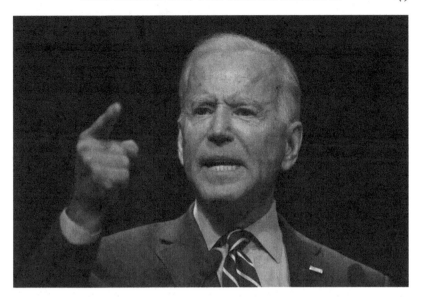

In his eighties, Joe Biden was the oldest president ever to occupy the White House.
(© *Gage Skidmore via Creative Commons*)

People aged sixty-five and up already form the biggest voting bloc in most states. Between now and 2040, the senior population is projected to swell by 44 percent while the eighteen-to-sixty-four population grows by just 6 percent. And many of those elders will have no qualms about keeping older politicians in office. As New York City mayor Eric Adams notes: People on social media don't choose candidates—people on Social Security do.

Biden's decision to abandon his 2024 reelection campaign capped a spirited national debate over how old is too old to serve as the nation's chief executive. The voting public seems split over whether that's a legitimate concern or antiquated thinking.

Norm Abelson, a ninety-plus-year-old journalist, memoirist, columnist, and poet who lives in Maine—demographically the oldest US state—suggests the debate is misdirected. Instead, he poses an alternative question: How young is too young to take on what well could be the toughest job on Earth?

"There's an African saying," he writes. "'When an old man dies, a library burns down.' When I was a kid, my parents told me that when an older person entered the room I was to stand as a show of respect. It isn't that all of us older people are smarter, but rather it's that the very experience of living, with all its bumps and setbacks, provides balance and perspective. It gives the opportunity to learn from mistakes, to grow and mature."

Abelson adds: "The Constitution sets thirty-five as the minimum age for accession to the presidency. It wisely does not set a maximum. Being in one's latter years hardly disqualifies a person to lead. And neither does being young necessarily make one a better candidate to occupy the Oval Office or any other responsible position. The measure shouldn't be whether one lives long enough to finish a term; it should be what people are able to accomplish, and the grace of their leadership, in whatever time on Earth they are given."

Politicians used to kiss babies to curry favor among young families and win votes. In our centenarian future, given the increasing political clout of super-agers, they'll likely need to lavish their attention and affection on elders.

Others, though, are asking equally ponderous questions about the ethics of electing very old leaders—questions that not only concern their real or perceived cognitive capabilities, but the consequences of the subsequent muting, intentional or not, of younger perspectives.

In Congress, boomers and the Silent Generation long have had a nearly implacable perch atop the influence pyramid. Viewed from the perspective of millennials and members of Generation Z, most senior US officials are antiques. Left to their own devices, some of these politicians seem determined to equal the granddaddy of them all: Senator Strom Thurmond of South Carolina, who was barely six months into retirement when he died at 100.

Senate Republican leader Mitch McConnell, like Biden, is in his eighties. Iowa senator Chuck Grassley, just reelected, will be ninety-five when he completes his eighth term. The late California senator Dianne Feinstein, who still held office when she died at ninety, decided not to seek reelection in 2024 amid mounting concerns about her cognitive health and memory. All told, one in four members of Congress is older than seventy—the oldest both chambers have ever been, marking the peak, so far, of a trend that began in the 1990s. The 2022 midterms injected incrementally more youth, lowering federal lawmakers' median age from 61.7 to 59.2. But their ages still don't mesh well with America's demographics: While half of the nation is under the age of forty, only 5 percent of Congress is.

"Not too long from now, many of these fine people will be incapacitated or dead. Who will take charge then, if younger people have not been brought in and prepared?" asks Katha Pollitt, a columnist for *The Nation*. "And by younger, I don't mean sixty-somethings. Half the US population is under forty. With the best will in the world, someone born during the Truman administration can barely grasp what life is like for them."

The United States isn't alone in this regard. Queen Elizabeth II, Britain's longest-reigning monarch, held the throne for seventy years before her death at ninety-six; her son and successor, King Charles III, is in his mid-seventies. Two-time Malaysian prime minister Mahathir Mohamad, who became the world's oldest leader at ninety-two, mounted a reelection bid at ninety-seven. Brazil's new president, Luiz Inácio Lula da Silva, is approaching eighty. And, like the United States, the world's other superpowers are in seniors' hands: Indian prime minister Narendra Modi, Russian leader Vladimir Putin, and Chinese president Xi Jinping are all in their seventies.

Interestingly, Europe, demographically the world's oldest continent, has been electing a crop of young leaders in their thirties and forties in recent years, reversing a time-honored tradition of letting the very old stay in charge until they run out of gas. Winston Churchill didn't resign as Britain's prime minister until he was eighty, and France's Charles de Gaulle until he was seventy-nine. Konrad Adenauer, Germany's first postwar leader, was eighty-seven when he finally stepped down as chancellor and remained head of the ruling Christian Democratic Union until a year before his death at ninety-one. Men for all seasons, their fortitude and faculties nonetheless differed: Adenauer exhibited mental sharpness to the end, while Churchill suffered from mild but progressive dementia in his later years.

If it intruded at all on the curmudgeonly prime minister while he was still in office—the International Churchill Society insists it did not—he maintained an uncompromised ability to deliver a withering zinger with flawless comic timing. Biographers say the 2017 biopic *Darkest Hour* got it right when it portrayed an awkward exchange between Churchill and an aide who knocked on a lavatory door to relay a message from a high-ranking British government officer. Here's Churchill, played by Gary Oldman in an Academy Award–winning performance, sitting on a toilet in the House of Commons:

> Please tell the Privy Seal that I'm sealed in the privy and I can only deal with one shit at a time.

Churchill was already an old man, and Elizabeth still a young woman, when the statesman and the sovereign first tangled. Eventually, though, the queen came to greatly admire Churchill, delivering a touching final tribute as he approached the end of his life. Both extremes in the evolution of their relationship—Elizabeth as she initially bristled at their generation gap, and later, after she bridged it—are poignantly showcased in the popular Netflix dramatic series *The Crown*:

(Elizabeth) I would ask you to consider your response in light of the respect that my rank and office deserve, not that which my age and gender might suggest.

[And some years later . . .]

(Elizabeth) Where would Great Britain be without its greatest Briton? God bless you, Winston.

Europe's shift to Gen X leaders may have helped keep the continent innovative while avoiding political impotence and economic collapse. An exhaustive study of seven European countries—Denmark, Finland, France, Italy, Germany, the Netherlands, and the United Kingdom—led by Vincenzo Atella and Lorenzo Carbonari of the University of Rome and published in the *Journal of Applied Economics* finds that gerontocracies trail nations with younger, more nimble leadership when it comes to economic growth. Why? Because their political and economic elites tend not only to maintain things as they are, the researchers say, but consistently demonstrate an inability to seize the opportunity offered by new technologies and make the best long-term choices for the economy as a whole:

"Over the last three decades, many European economies have fallen into an old-age trap, a self-reinforcing mechanism whereby elites, generally the most aged individuals, have used control of the political system to exclude new generations, who are reasonably the most dynamic and innovative part of the population, from access to power."

Their conclusion: "When relatively young people cease to be the engine of an economy, long-run economic growth is endangered." (They also get a dig in about older leaders' "obsolescence." Ouch.)

What can result—especially in places like Europe, where low birth rates tip the scales in favor of older citizens, further enhancing their power—isn't just economic stagnation but potentially something far more consequential: political instability.

"There are concerns about elderly and long-serving leaders," says Thomas Klassen, a professor at the School of Public Policy & Administration at Canada's York University. He worries that aging superpower leaders represent a serious threat to the world order because, in their determination to cling to power, they rarely have succession plans that will ensure a peaceful transition when the time comes.

And they're detached from the masses in other ways.

"They may be out of touch with the younger generations they need to represent," Klassen writes in a commentary for *The Conversation*. "Solutions to policy conundrums that worked for them decades ago might no longer apply now or in the future. Their attitudes and perspectives may become conservative or inflexible. . . . They probably don't have children in kindergarten and so don't see how policy plays out in real life."

Bucking the trend is Nancy Pelosi. At eighty-two, and arguably at the top of her game, the Democrat nobly decided to step down as House Speaker and let a new generation rise. With that, the torch passed swiftly to a man three decades younger than she: Representative Hakeem Jeffries of New York, the first Black person to head a major political party in Congress.

"She has now had the courage to step back, making way for new leaders and new ideas," says Gerald Warburg, a professor of public policy at the University of Virginia.

Younger generations have been restive, to say the least.

Those contemptuous "Okay boomer" memes that have gone viral on TikTok and other social platforms over the past few years didn't just spring up out of the ether. They reflect deep-seated frustrations that millennials and Gen Zers feel when they encounter many older Americans' smug financial security and perceived passivity on existential crises like climate change. And let's face it: Boomers who dare to diss piercings or body art while wearing dad jeans or Capri pants only widen the generation gap and inflame the culture wars. (Aside to my fellow boomers: Sorry, but what the hell happened to us? Have we forgotten our own anti-establishment protests and the countercultures we so raucously established in the sixties and seventies? Some of us deserve to be pricked hard with the pins on our rusty "Don't Trust Anyone Over 30" buttons.)

One consequence of older leadership is that it risks prioritizing seniors' issues and concerns over those of younger citizens. Granted, that may become less problematic as the population ages more profoundly, but for now, people in their teens to their forties rightfully may worry they're being neglected.

Lawmakers in a gerontocracy, some caution, tend to devote more time and resources to shoring up Social Security funding and Medicare entitlements than addressing the skyrocketing cost of rents and college educations. "The age of those holding executive, legislative, and judicial power in Washington, DC, sends a warning," says York University's Klassen. "American politicians are much more generous to the old than they are to the young. After all, the country does have [universal] public health care, but only for those sixty-five and older."

AARP alone has 38 million members, which gives it considerable leverage as it lobbies Capitol Hill and makes its presence known in all fifty statehouses. "The clout of older voters continues to grow," says Cristina Martin Firvida, the organization's chief of governmental affairs. But, she reminds me, they don't all speak with one voice: "Older voters are not homogenous. They don't all want the same things. They don't all look the same. They don't all live in the same places."

Prophets of doom envision that all this senior influence peddling will come at a terrible cost, deepening intergenerational conflict as the young chafe beneath the suffocating dominance of elders who refuse to step aside. Add persistent racial and economic disparities in who gets access to clean food, health care, and the levers of power, they warn, and we've got a combustive mix with the potential to unleash social upheaval on a scale we've never seen.

Sociologist Beth Truesdale of Michigan's W.E. Upjohn Institute believes such concerns are overblown.

"I think the evidence suggests that's a misapprehension. Places that do better by their older adults also tend to do better by their younger adults and by their children," Truesdale tells me. The trick, she says, is to build a society that allows people to live their best lives at every age.

"I don't think people need to worry that an aging population means the young ones get less," she says. "But the longer we wait, the more expensive it gets. We need to be putting policies in place to support people who are older now and who are retired. But we also need to be making investments now in the people who are middle-aged and younger, because relatively small investments now can lead to big payoffs later."

There's no denying one dynamic, though: Older voters overwhelmingly tend to support candidates who look like them: old (sorry, "experienced"—code for the same thing). Meanwhile, more than 70 percent of eligible voters aged sixty and up cast ballots in presidential elections; fewer than 50 percent of those aged eighteen to twenty-nine vote.

The strong and decisive turnout of millennial and Gen Z voters in the 2022 midterms is a bright spot in an otherwise bleak picture. Younger voters played a key role in battleground states— Florida, Georgia, Michigan, North Carolina, New Hampshire, Nevada, Ohio, Pennsylvania, and Wisconsin—helping Democrats keep the US Senate and hold Republican gains in the House to a minimum. In Michigan, some stood in line until 2:00 a.m. to cast their ballots. In Florida, they elected the first Gen Z member of Congress: twenty-five-year-old Maxwell Alejandro Frost, a Democrat who tweeted after his historic win: "Don't count young people out."

Cristina Tzintzún Ramirez, president of NextGen, a progressive youth advocacy nonprofit and political action committee, tells *The Guardian* that voters in their late teens, twenties, and thirties frequently are labeled as apathetic when they actually constitute the most politically engaged subset of the US electorate. "They're voting more. They're participating in protests. They are more avid readers of politics and social issues," she says.

And by overwhelmingly supporting Democrats and progressive causes, they function as a foil to aging conservatives—particularly fifty- and sixty-something white evangelicals—who embrace Trump and his baseless claims of a leftist conspiracy to rig and steal elections. (Overall, the Pew Research Center says, older Americans vote predominantly Republican and their younger counterparts lean Democratic. There are, of course, plenty of exceptions—retirees who backed Bernie and Biden, and Turning Point USA–type conservatives in their twenties and thirties who tracked with Trump; Florida governor Ron DeSantis; or Nikki Haley, former US ambassador to the United Nations.)

John Della Volpe, director of polling at the Harvard Kennedy School's Institute of Politics, believes voters aged eighteen to twenty-nine are playing an increasingly decisive role in presidential elections. If you're running for higher office, he says, you ignore them at your peril: "Many of the young men and women who voted for Democrats [in 2022] have a complicated relationship with America. They have been told of our exceptionalism but rarely experienced it themselves or seen our nation united."

Evoking shades of Volpe, New York representative Alexandria Ocasio-Cortez, a member of the progressive Squad in Congress, tweets: "By 2024, Millennials & Gen Z voters will outnumber voters who are baby boomers and older, 45/25. We are beginning to see the political impacts of that generational shift."

Senator Bernie Sanders, another darling of the left, agrees: "Without the major turnout of younger voters, we would have seen a very different outcome. . . . But now I am asking the younger generations: Continue to stay engaged in the struggle."

Sanders, of course, is that notable exception in America's aging political elite: He's in his early eighties, with wispy white hair and a grouchy demeanor, yet as a socialist independent is beloved by voters a quarter of his age who are young enough to be his grandkids. He and Senator Elizabeth Warren of Massachusetts have championed the issues younger voters consistently identify as most important to them: climate change, relief from crushing student loan debt, abortion rights, and a level financial playing field for everyone, not just the rich. (Seventy-six percent of Gen Z voters surveyed after the 2022 midterms by the education advocacy organization Murmuration, the Walton Family Foundation, and the public opinion firm SocialSphere said preserving women's reproductive rights was among their top issues; 73 percent also cited climate change; and 72 percent pointed to student loan debt relief.)

Sanders's relentless and bombastic challenges to the status quo have made him a counterculture icon—an unlikely yet larger-than-life, working-class hero. "If other Democrats want to be as popular with Generation Z as Sanders is, they'll have to start incorporating some of his strategies into their own campaigns," says Jack Kapcar, a University of Michigan student journalist.

As encouraging as young voters' growing political awareness is, don't look for elders to cede the public square for another three or four decades, when the last of the outsized baby boom generation are gone, setting the stage for a brief but turbulent population nosedive. It won't last long; in the United States, Gen Xers will take the baton for a time before handing it off to the millennials, who at 72 million strong already have surpassed boomers as the nation's largest living adult generation.

If anything, there are signs that senior activists are upping their game and taking to the streets. Th!rd Act, a new organization that's "building a community of Americans over the age of sixty determined to change the world for the better," is mobilizing retirees and others to join protests and demonstrations promoting progressive causes ranging from a campaign for a sustainable society and planet to an intergenerational movement aimed at transforming how Wall Street and Washington function. Some of its members are veterans of the 1960s civil rights and antiwar struggles returning, in a way, to their radical roots. Others are newbies who've never marched, chanted, or waved a sign. Now you'll find them out there holding placards with slogans like "Old & Bold" and "No Time to Waste."

"We're used to thinking that humans grow more conservative as they age, perhaps because we have more to protect, or simply because we're used to things the way they are," its website says. "But our generations saw enormous positive change early in our lives—the civil rights movement, for instance, or the fight to end massive wars or guarantee the rights of women. And now we fear that the promise of those changes may be dying, as the planet heats and inequality grows." In its optimism, the group doesn't mention how old and powerful conservative forces have reshaped the Supreme Court, or the fallout of that: the overturning of the 1973 *Roe v. Wade* decision guaranteeing a constitutional right to an abortion, and a growing sense that affirmative action policies aimed at improving employment and educational opportunities for members of minority groups could be next.

Th!rd Act, which uses the terms "Experienced Americans" and "Third Actors" to describe the 10,000 people who daily turn sixty in the United States, insists institutions can't and won't ignore boomers who identify as change agents. Why not? "Because we vote and because we have a large—maybe an overlarge—share of the country's assets. And many of us have kids and grandkids and great-grandkids: We have, in other words, very real reasons to worry and to work."

In a video aired on PBS, Th!rd Act's founder, environmentalist Bill McKibben, says his generation has a pivotal role to play in combating climate change. "It helps to have some people with hairlines like mine engaged in this work," he says, and elaborates:

> It must be said, kids are doing extraordinary work organizing around climate change, but there is something a little undignified about taking the biggest problem that the world's ever gotten into and asking junior high school students to solve it for you. . . .
>
> If you're in your sixties or seventies or eighties, your first act was in that period of rapid social, cultural, political transformation of the sixties and seventies. Our second act was a little more about consumerism than it was about citizenship. That's water under the bridge. Now people emerge in their third act with skills, resources, with time, which they may not have had before, and with kids or grandkids. I mean, your legacy is the planet you leave behind for the people you love the most.
>
> And the planet we're going to leave behind and the democracy we're going to leave behind at the moment seem likely to be much shabbier than the ones we were born into. Most older people realize that, and that there's real meaning in continuing to try the project of building a better society.

It's a refreshing and hopeful perspective, considering the dystopian handwringing you'll still occasionally encounter about elders taking up space and depleting resources. Over the years, Orwellian attitudes about seniors' place in society have led to some spectacularly unfortunate bluster, and from both ends of the political spectrum.

In 1984, when he was still in his forties, Colorado's late Democratic governor Dick Lamm caused an uproar by saying publicly he thought elderly people who are terminally ill have "a duty to die and get out of the way" rather than prolong their lives through artificial means. Conveniently for Lamm, he ended up living to eighty-five.

More recently, in the early days of the coronavirus pandemic, Texas's then sixty-nine-year-old Republican lieutenant governor, Dan Patrick, reaped a whirlwind of his own by insisting grandparents like him would rather sacrifice themselves and die of COVID-19 than imperil the economy for their grandchildren by not working. Patrick suggested shutdowns should be avoided at all costs, even if it cost some people their lives. He was tragically right about that last bit: COVID-19, of course, exacted a horribly disproportionate toll on people aged sixty-five and older.

Not to give this particular purveyor of pap needless oxygen, but lest you're unaware of the toxic disdain for our elders that's being spewed by some on the right, conservative millennial pundit Julius Krein floats an indecent proposal: "Higher tax rates should be imposed on anyone who continues to work full time or hold 'systemically important' positions after age sixty-five, and those over seventy should be automatically forced into retirement where they belong. The elderly can still serve as part-time advisers, freelance writers, and so on, but they should not hold important positions. Current political officeholders over the age of seventy should have the good sense to resign, and the Constitution should be amended to include maximum ages in addition to minimums."

Krein could have learned a thing or two from the celebrated *New Yorker* cartoonist Jean-Jacques Sempé, who died at eighty-nine in his beloved Provence after a stroke robbed him of his speech but not his piercing intellect. I regret that I never met Sempé myself, but a touching tribute by a mutual friend, journalist and author Mort Rosenblum, makes me feel as though I did:

"These days, I think a lot about age, the passage of time and how things are changing so fast around us. Young people who grow up in a warp-speed interconnected world tend to dismiss elders as clueless relics who should be moved aside simply on principle. Sitting there with Jean-Jacques, sharp as ever but physically silenced, I saw what a folly that is. His gift for picking up nuanced details sharpened over time, and his lived experience shaped an uncommon grasp of the human condition. Age is luck of the draw. At some point, it gets us all. But until it does, we can learn an awful lot from what lives well lived can teach us."

If aging America needs a new anthem, I nominate Neil Young's "Old Man":

Old man, look at my life
I'm a lot like you were.

THERE'S ANOTHER POTENTIAL DRAWBACK TO HAVING THE VERY OLD lead us: Statistically, they're far more likely to die in office.

We elect individuals, though, not statistical averages. Until recently, seniors like Biden and Trump showed they had sufficient mental and physical stamina to handle the rigors of the presidency—a pursuit that political strategist David Axelrod has called "a monstrously taxing job." And like it or not, one of the nation's most prominent longevity experts thinks both men have the potential to become super-agers.

S. Jay Olshansky, the University of Illinois epidemiologist we met in chapter 1, has extensively studied US presidents and their ages.

"Despite the science, the candidates themselves and their campaigns are still trying to weaponize age," he says.

Irking some older voters, Haley, who is fifty-two, capitalized on grave and widely held concerns about Biden's age with an opening presidential campaign pitch calling for mandatory mental competency tests for politicians older than seventy-five. Critics have denounced the proposal as blatantly ageist, and political analysts see it as a slight not only of Biden but of Trump, Haley's mentor and former boss.

Age has been red meat in American partisan politics for decades. In 1984, President Ronald Reagan, then seventy-three, famously was asked about his advanced years during a nationally televised debate with his Democratic opponent, Walter Mondale, then fifty-six. Reagan's response: "I want you to know that also I will not make age an issue of this campaign. I am not going to exploit, for political purposes, my opponent's youth and inexperience." The crowd burst into laughter; even Mondale cracked up; and a nation was charmed into submission. Just like Reagan himself, the outcome was straight out of Hollywood: He won another one for the Gipper with the biggest landslide in US history.

Five years after leaving office, Reagan publicly announced he had Alzheimer's disease. Close advisers already had said he seemed foggy at times in his second term, and although there's never been any evidence to suggest his cognitive functions were impaired during his presidency, all of us experience brain degradation. Our brains start shrinking in our thirties and forties, and by the time we're in our sixties, researchers say, the rate of shrinkage increases even more. Brain volume overall decreases with age, but particularly the size of our frontal lobes and hippocampus—specific regions of the brain responsible for cognitive function. Our cerebral cortex also thins, which slows our thought process and decision-making, and neurons begin to die off. Along the way, memory and the ability to multitask take a hit.

As much as we want to believe age is just a number, it clearly isn't. Biologically, chemically, and psychologically, we're not the same at eighty as we are at forty-five. None of this stops older politicians seen as long in the tooth from having a little fun at their own expense.

Trailing Democrat Barack Obama in the polls a few days before the 2008 presidential election, Republican senator John McCain acknowledged the elephant in the room during an appearance on *Saturday Night Live.* "Good evening, my fellow Americans," the seventy-two-year-old said. "I ask you, what should we be looking for in our next president? Certainly, someone who is very, very, very old." A year earlier, while campaigning in New Hampshire, McCain touted his stamina when a high school student questioned his age, then delivered this mock rebuke: "Thanks for the question, you little jerk. You're drafted."

There's no substitute for experience. Yet there are persuasive arguments for standing down and giving way.

Peter Suderman, an editor at *Reason*, bemoans "the general lack of fresh thinking in politics."

"When someone has been in the same role for decades, they tend to fall back on old habits, and it shows," he says. "Biden first entered the Senate in 1973. Pelosi has been in Congress since 1987. There's a reason that American politics today feels so bereft of new ideas: Too many of the people at the top pretty clearly haven't had one in a very long time."

Paul Irving, a senior fellow at the nonpartisan Milken Institute think tank and a leading expert on longevity and our rapidly changing demographics, acknowledges the narrative: "There is a point of view out there that US politics is dominated in both parties by septuagenarians and octogenarians and that the young people, as a result, aren't having an opportunity to emerge and grow." But Irving rejects the notion of age limits in politics out of hand despite widespread public support for the concept.

Ask him, though, if it's cool for older people to soldier on infinitely—so long as they've got the energy and the votes—and the question gives pause to the seventy-something founding chair of Milken's Center for the Future of Aging. Twice in his own life, Irving says, he's stepped away from a leadership role to empower a younger person to take over. That doesn't mean, he hastens to add, that he's kicked himself to the curb.

"I think we do need to be generous to younger people," he says. On the flip side, "I think we need to both seek and expect respect and dignity and the opportunity to remain involved. We need to be able to manifest our general inclination to pass down, pay forward, mentor. As I often say to people my age and older, despite the fact that we have a lot of differences in America, most of us who had good parents heard when we were growing up: 'Whatever you do in life, leave the world in a better place than you found it.' And I very much believe in that. I think the importance of older people investing in younger people not only serves younger people; it serves older people as well."

Older people don't just have political clout. They've also got considerable economic power.

AMERICANS LIVING SIGNIFICANTLY LONGER AND HEALTHIER LIVES will pump $7.1 trillion into the US economy alone over the next fifty years, simply because they'll purchase more goods and services, says Dana Goldman, a University of Southern California economist.

As we explored in chapter 5, boomers are living longer and working longer. The labor force participation rate of people aged seventy and above is about 9 percent, and it's expected to rise to about 16 percent by 2035. Financially, it's time to start thinking of our oldest people more as GDP engines and less as brakes on the system, and our years of extra life as a lucrative dividend for ourselves, our families, and the economy as a whole.

"We are working beyond our sixty-fifth year if we choose," notes William Beach, who stepped down in March 2023 as commissioner of the US Bureau of Labor Statistics. "Our health is declining with each year, but not declining with the speed at which it used to decline. We have more wealth. We have more income. We are healthier. We are more educated than any generation ever."

Underscoring seniors' spending power, Beach points to a somewhat obscure but illuminating statistic: per capita spending on entertainment—going out to see a movie or catch a concert, investing in home theater equipment, or buying a boat or a recreational vehicle—by those of us who are sixty-five or older. In 2021, it was nearly $3,000 per person—almost the same amount that was spent annually by people aged fifty-five to sixty-four, and substantially more than what twenty-five- to thirty-four-year-olds shelled out.

Consumers older than fifty control a staggering 83 percent of household wealth, says Joseph Coughlin, who runs the Massachusetts Institute of Technology's AgeLab and is the author of 2017's *The Longevity Economy*. Harley-Davidson's average buyer, he notes, is fifty, and the motorcycle manufacturer better known for catering to younger, more badass riders has been lowering seat heights so older customers with creaky joints can mount its bikes more easily.

By 2030, Coughlin says, the fifty-five-plus population will have driven 50 percent of US consumer spending growth since 2008; 67 percent of Japan's; and 86 percent of Germany's. "It's no exaggeration to say that the world's most advanced economies will soon revolve around the needs, wants, and whims of grandparents," he writes.

There's also a small but inspiring number of us who are still working deep into our nineties, if not beyond, at jobs we love.

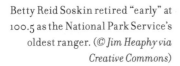

Betty Reid Soskin retired "early" at 100.5 as the National Park Service's oldest ranger. (© *Jim Heaphy via Creative Commons*)

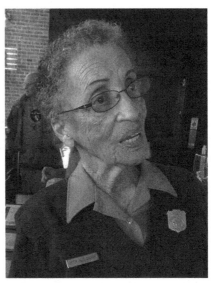

Take Betty Reid Soskin, who retired "early" as the National Park Service's oldest ranger at 100-and-a-half. A Black woman who came of age at a time when people of color were segregated from whites, Ranger Betty, as she's affectionately known, drew from her own rich personal history as she led public programs at the Rosie the Riveter World War II Home Front National Historical Park in Richmond, California, highlighting the experiences of Black Americans during the war. She started as a temp at age eighty-four. "It has proven to bring meaning to my final years," she says.

Or Brazil's Walter Orthmann, who didn't retire until age 102 at the textile company he joined as a fifteen-year-old shipping clerk. Orthmann, who rose to sales manager, became the Guinness World Record holder for longest career with the same company. "When we do what we like," he says, "we don't see the time go by."

One of the nation's most astonishing and inspiring examples of a very, very, *very* long career was that of US District Judge Wesley Brown, who died at 104 as the oldest sitting federal judge in American history. Sharp and competent to the end, with a wicked sense of humor—Brown used to warn lawyers gearing up for lengthy trials in his Kansas courtroom that he might not be alive for their closing arguments—he credited his very caseload for extending his life by keeping his mind and body active and giving him a sense of purpose. Well past his 100th birthday, he was still taking the stairs to his fourth-floor chambers. A year before his death, asked how he intended to leave the bench that President John F. Kennedy appointed him to in 1962, he quipped: "Feet first."

"As a federal judge, I was appointed for life or good behavior, whichever I lose first," he once told the Associated Press. "You got to have a reason to live. As long as you perform a public service, you have a reason to live."

We're all better acquainted with another exceptionally long-serving judge: US Supreme Court Justice Ruth Bader Ginsburg. She was still serving out her lifetime appointment when she died at eighty-seven. The acclaimed documentary *RBG*, released two years before her death in 2020, captures her vitality: lifting free weights in her office, signing autographs for adoring fans of the justice they'd nicknamed "The Notorious RBG," and breaking the internet each time she wrote a dissent. As Ginsburg drops to the gym floor to do some planks, one of two chuckling older admirers intones:

> I've heard she does twenty pushups three times a week or something. I mean, we can't even get off the floor. We can't even get *down* to the floor.

Social media influencer and fashionista Iris Apfel was like that. Apfel, who died at 102, sometimes gave the impression she was just getting started. Apfel liked to call herself "the world's oldest teenager," and her trademark oversized round glasses, flamboyant outfits, and irreverence gained her nearly two and a half million followers

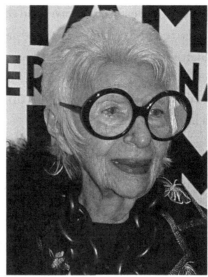

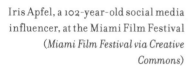

Iris Apfel, a 102-year-old social media influencer, at the Miami Film Festival (*Miami Film Festival via Creative Commons*)

on Instagram and numerous *Vogue, Vanity Fair,* and *Harper's Bazaar* covers. The style legend's cheeky catchphrase: "More is more & less is a bore." In 2018, she became the oldest person to have a Barbie doll created in her likeness.

"I don't look back," she told an interviewer in 2022. "The past is the past and it's finished. I don't dwell on it. And I don't do too much with the future because we don't know if we'll have one. So, I've learned to live in the now."

Seniors are wielding their influence well beyond politics and economics. In their millions, they are volunteering and committing random acts of philanthropy, forming the vanguard of a vast corps of people who are giving back in innumerable ways. As their life spans stretch beyond 100, look for their good works to multiply exponentially.

Experience Corps, a program run by the AARP Foundation, places volunteers aged fifty and up in schools to serve as tutors helping students improve their reading skills by the time they complete the third grade. Organizers call it a triple win because it helps students succeed, older adults thrive, and communities flourish. Linda Fong, a retired civil engineer whose parents immigrated to the United States from China, says she's overjoyed to help non-native-speaking children master English. "Even more meaningful is knowing that I've created a connection with this future generation," she adds in a blog post.

Along the way, volunteers like Fong are adding to the length and vibrancy of their already extending lives. Research by AmeriCorps, an independent agency of the US government that mobilizes more than 5 million volunteers, finds people who donate their time and talents have lower mortality rates, greater functional ability, and lower rates of depression later in life than those who don't. Those health benefits are greater for volunteers who are sixty and older: They tend to suffer fewer cardiovascular, cognitive, and pulmonary problems, and have a reduced risk of developing crippling osteoarthritis.

"Aging is not an inevitable period of decline. Older people make multiple contributions to society that in fact outweigh the costs that society has to bear," says John Beard, a former World Health Organization official who now directs the International Longevity Center-USA at Columbia University.

It's probably a long shot, but if seniors stay engaged like this, maybe the United States finally will amass the political will needed to catch up with countries it badly lags—like Germany, Japan, and South Korea—in establishing a nationally insured elder care system.

Elders in those nations don't bankrupt themselves when they reach a point where they need care. Americans do: routinely, tragically, and most maddening of all, avoidably.

"In the United States at the moment, this is done very badly," says Beard, an Australian who takes a dim view of American exceptionalism. How can we crow and preen when Medicare doesn't cover the cost of nursing home care? And when people in their prime earning years have to exit the workforce to attend to their aging and ailing parents, compromising their own future financial security in the process?

I can already hear neoconservatives and nationalists jeering, "Love it or leave it!" Here's a more patriotic thought: How about love it and fix it?

"Why are we willing to spend on a BMW and support the car industry or whatever other industries government supports in one way or another, but we don't do it for the care industry when the care economy is enormous?" Beard asks. In the United States, we impose on needy elders our cultural imperative of individualism and its cruel (in this context) edict that everybody must take personal responsibility for themselves. In Europe, with its more social orientation, there's a conviction that society bears some responsibility and government can provide ways to absorb the costs.

"You just don't have that in the US," Beard tells me. "And you know, we talk about it and I don't understand why people just immediately shut down. They can't even listen to the arguments."

As we'll see in the next chapter, we literally cannot afford to ignore what's broken any longer.

Whether we end up making it to 78.1, Biden's age when he was sworn in, or 108.1, our quality of life—if not our very lives themselves—will depend on what we do, and don't do, in the next few years.

CHAPTER NINE

WHO WILL CARE FOR US?
AND WHO WILL PAY?

How do you feel about a robot taking care of you when you're 100? Because it's going to be a hard "no" for me.

But with so many of us living longer and eventually needing care, it's inevitable that artificial intelligence will be pressed into service to help, in ways at once enthralling and terrifying. It's already happening.

What's currently creeping me out is Miroki, a vaguely feline, quasi-elfin robot that France-based Enchanted Tools has designed to deliver food trays and cups of water to hospitalized patients, freeing up staff to perform more health care–specific tasks. He? She? It? has been endowed with a whimsical personality inspired by a mashup of anime films. Part Sonic the Hedgehog and part Link from Nintendo's *The Legend of Zelda*, Miroki stands a little over three feet (one meter) tall and rolls around on a large gyroscopic sphere. It's capable of interactive expressions with its disproportionately large eyes that crinkle along with a smile or widen like they're about to well up with tears, depending on the responding patient's facial expression or tone of voice.

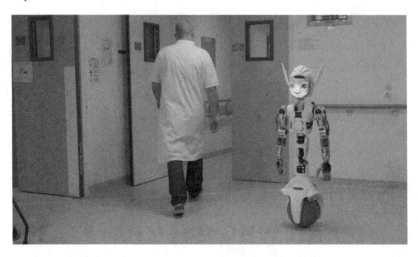

Miroki, a robot developed by France-based Enchanted Tools, awaits orders at Broca Hospital. (*Enchanted Tools/BrocaLab*)

Chances are you're nowhere near as neurotic as I am and would find Miroki impossibly endearing. That's what Enchanted Tools founder and CEO Jérôme Monceaux is counting on as he develops a line of semi-humanoid robots he hopes we'll find engaging and approachable. (Pepper, another of Monceaux's android creations done while he was with Aldebaran, a robotics competitor he cofounded, cracks dad jokes to seniors while it's reminding them to eat, exercise, or take their meds: "I went on a date with a Roomba last week. It totally sucked.") Personally, I'd feel more comfortable locked alone in an attic filled with M3GAN dolls and circus clowns, but hey, that's just me.

Two things, though, in defense of the industry: Dreamers like Monceaux are adhering—so far, anyway—to a strict code of ethics that forbids them from ever engineering a robot to dominate a human. And at least they're thinking creatively, if unconventionally, about the caregiving question confronting humanity.

We're in the throes of a crisis, and the consequences can be beyond dire for our most venerable and vulnerable citizens. What could possibly go wrong? A lot, as it turns out. To paraphrase Shakespeare's *Julius Caesar*, the fault is not in our machines, but in ourselves.

And no one should ever have to make choices like those that confronted 108-year-old Juliet Bernstein.

MENTALLY SHARP BUT PHYSICALLY FRAIL, BERNSTEIN, A long-retired New York City schoolteacher, launched a crowd-funding campaign so she could avoid an impersonal death in the relative anonymity of a nursing facility and instead live out her days in her cozy Cape Cod, Massachusetts, home. "I saw it was being done for someone whose child was very sick," she told the *Boston Globe*. "So I said, 'I'm not going to go to a nursing home. I'm remaining here.'"

It worked out for Bernstein in the end—she died there on her own terms after raising more than $130,000 to pay for home health care attendants. But is society really going to normalize this kind of Hail Mary, *Hunger Games*–esque desperation play, where our future well-being rises and falls on which causes-célèbres get traction on social media?

As grim as that sounds, we're likely to see more of our grand-mothers and grandfathers take to GoFundMe. Many have limited options: Medicare doesn't pay for extended nursing home care, and assisted living facilities are outrageously expensive. In the United States, the national assisted-living average is just over $4,000 a month, but that can range from $3,000 in Georgia to nearly twice that in New Jersey. It's so expensive, the average person must save 7.5 percent of their income for a decade to afford assisted living if they'll eventually need it. Meanwhile, in the United States, we're going backward, not forward, with our federal government cutting Medicare payments to doctors.

To call caregiving in the United States broken is a bit misleading. Brokenness implies that something was working and it ceased to function, and America's elder care system arguably has never worked.

It's not just an American problem. In Britain, the Royal College of Physicians warns that a drastic shortage of doctors with special training to attend to the largest generation of elderly adults in human history means the United Kingdom is "sleepwalking into an avoidable crisis of care for older people."

The coming rise of centenarians will test nations' long-term care systems in unprecedented ways, but we're unprepared, even though neon warning signs are blinking all around us.

In the United States, elder care is busting Medicare and Medicaid budgets. Who picks up the slack if boomers, and the Gen Xers right behind them, fall short in preparing financially and exhaust their limited resources? The future for subsequent waves of centenarians looks unappealing: Millennials, Gen Zers, and Alphas could be called on to care for their 100-year-old elders, but with far less to work with, even as they continue their own march to 100—all while coping with the worst that climate change has in store.

"The real risk America faces with centenarians is ignoring the message in the numbers," analyst Chris Farrell says. Translation, with apologies to The Beatles:

Will you still need me
Will you still feed me
When I'm 104?

The very bones and viscera of modern society are about to be rearranged, and it's all just around the corner. Having overcome so much over the millennia to be in a position to live so incredibly long, we've got to get this right. Will we have the courage and resolve to act?

Our next steps are critical. They'll determine whether we live long and prosper—or live long as paupers.

UNDERSCORING WHAT WE'RE UP AGAINST: JUST A DECADE AGO, something called the "caregiver support ratio"—the number of people aged forty-five to sixty-four available to care for people aged eighty and older—was seven to one. By 2030, it's forecast to drop to four to one, and by 2050, to three to one, meaning there will be alarmingly fewer younger people to help feed, bathe, and dress us.

There's a simple explanation: The boomers are getting older. In this decade, the oldest of them will be in their eighties, and by 2050, the youngest of them will be there. In a few short years, boomers will go from providing care to needing it.

An estimated 53 million Americans are serving as family caregivers and spending an average of 26 percent of their household income taking care of loved ones. There's an impression that the vast majority of caregivers are women, but four in ten are men. A quarter of all caregivers are millennials or Gen Zers and care for more than one person, juggling their time and attention between a child and a grandparent or someone else who's disabled.

Debra Whitman, AARP's policy chief, calls them "the invisible army."

When I talked to Whitman, she'd just returned from New Zealand, where average life expectancy exceeds America's by three full years. Granted, it's a small nation—in comparison, there are 38 million AARP members alone and only 5 million Kiwis total— but New Zealand managed to map out a plan ensuring that as its citizens age, they'll have care that's not just adequate but culturally appropriate for its indigenous Māori communities, including government-funded, in-home support. "When I go to other countries," she says, "those that have plans for an aging population do much better than countries like ours that seem to have not noticed we have an aging population and have no plan for it."

Jason Resendez, president and CEO of the National Alliance for Caregiving, calls caregivers "invisible philanthropists" who offer society their time and talents rather than wealth. They also sacrifice earnings: Lost income due to family caregiving is estimated at $522 billion each year.

"Like the working poor, America's 53 million family caregivers are often unseen and undervalued," Resendez says. "Care has consequences. They come in the form of poorer health outcomes for caregivers, and they come in the form of economic instability."

Catherine Collinson, president and CEO of the Transamerica Center for Retirement Studies, took some time off to care for an aging parent. She thought it would be a few months. It ended up being five years. "We don't know how long the duties will last. Months can turn into years," she says, adding something else she's learned the hard way through personal experience: It can be very difficult to reenter the workforce. Her research shows eight in ten family caregivers end up making some kind of adjustment to their work situations. Many miss workdays. Others take leaves of absence. And some quit their jobs altogether.

"Family caregiving is a huge bite out of somebody's pocket," says John Schall, CEO of the Caregiver Action Network, who notes that the average household spends between $7,000 and $10,000 a year on it when the median US annual income hovers around $60,000. He and others are pressing Congress to enact a $5,000 federal tax write-off for people engaged as caregivers. They also want lawmakers to consider giving Social Security credits to people who must leave the workforce to provide care, so there are no gaps in their earnings records, and they don't end up financially compromised when they eventually retire.

Women, a slim majority of all caregivers, are particularly affected, says Yulya Truskinovsky, an assistant professor of economics at

Wayne State University in Detroit who has studied the impacts of family caregiving on the economy. "For them, earnings and labor force participation peak in their mid- to late-fifties. So, when they take on these caregiving roles, it's exactly when they're hitting peak earnings to set them up for their financial future."

In the United States, informal caregivers' combined contributions to a part of the economy that's largely unseen are mind-boggling: One in five Americans does this essential work for a family member, devoting 340 billion hours a year to it, collectively, and all for free. The estimated annual economic value of their unpaid contributions? A whopping $470 billion. That's $100 billion more than all out-of-pocket spending on health care in 2017, and $40 billion more than the total value of the agriculture, forestry, and mining sectors combined.

Meanwhile, Americans aged sixty-five and older now outnumber those fifty and younger, a trend that's only going to become more pronounced as fertility decreases and childbirths decline. By 2050, researchers say, people who are fifty-plus will comprise 27 percent of the US population. Something similar is happening in other rapidly graying societies: That same year, 40 percent of the populations of both Germany and Japan will be older than sixty-five.

Here's how those two countries differ from the United States, though: They have universal systems funding mandatory long-term care insurance for their populations—programs that cover the costs of both institutional and home care. South Korea has had a program like that since 2008. Inexplicably, the United States, for all its wealth, does not.

"In many ways, the United States is an anomaly," says John Beard, the International Longevity Center-USA director. "I don't want to be overly critical, but you're the richest country in the world, and yet the poorest people in your country have so many adverse outcomes and shorter life spans. It's easy to look at the averages. And even on average, you don't do that well. If your median is worse than the global average, then what about what's happening with the other halves? Because they must be much worse."

Beard challenges the notion that a German, Japanese, or Korean approach is too expensive. The cost in Germany and Japan of paying for seniors' long-term care is about 3 percent of gross domestic product, "which is affordable when you consider the United States spends about 9 or 10 percent more on GDP for health care than other countries."

Korea's $5 billion a year long-term care insurance system puts America's feeble efforts to shame. It provides both institutional and home care with a maximum $1,300 annual copay, including mobile bathing units that help older adults in rural areas with toileting, and short-term, twenty-four-hour "respite care" that ensures aging loved ones are looked after for up to nine days a month so their caregivers can deal with business trips and other life interruptions. One complication: The country's birth rate, one of the lowest in all of Asia, could make it difficult to pay for this care in the years to come, says Jongseong Lee, deputy director of Korea's national Ministry of Health and Welfare and an architect of the program. "My biggest concern is its sustainability," he tells me.

The argument for taking a trans-societal approach in the United States has never been greater. Admittedly, it's an uphill battle in an individualistic country where pride in pulling ourselves up by our bootstraps is encoded into our collective DNA, and where many people condemn anything policy-wise that smacks of socialism. But our current system isn't cutting it—a damning assessment by the National Academies of Sciences, Engineering, and Medicine calls it "ineffective, inefficient, fragmented"—so, why not learn from other nations who've succeeded where we've failed? As the slain 1960s civil rights leader Malcolm X once said: "When 'I' is replaced by 'we,' even illness becomes wellness."

Meanwhile, that seismic demographic shift—more of us who are old, fewer of us who are young—is setting up a perfect caregiving storm, warns Linda Fried, dean of Columbia University's Mailman School of Public Health and a leader in the field of geriatric medicine.

"Who will care for older adults when there are fewer younger people?" she asks. "We're looking at a tsunami of needs. . . . We need each other across generations. We need to redesign, design anew, for a society we never had before: a society of longer lives."

The Stanford Center on Longevity also is sounding a clarion call to action: We must, it urges, "change the trajectory of aging and associated costs by starting now to redesign institutions, practices, and norms so that they align with today's reality" rather than that of the last century.

As the late US first lady Rosalynn Carter put it: "There are only four kinds of people in the world—those who have been caregivers, those who are currently caregivers, those who will be caregivers, and those who will need caregivers."

CARING FOR FAMILY MEMBERS HAS ALWAYS BEEN FRAUGHT.
Many of us are looking after our elders even as we're working full-time and raising our kids. But the care itself also has become much more complicated. Caregivers who have little or no training increasingly are finding themselves dealing with not only their own chronic physical infirmities but their emotional difficulties, too. Sixty percent care for someone with Alzheimer's or another form of dementia. And one in three is doing all of that with no help from anyone else, many forgoing their own health and emotional needs, the National Alliance for Caregiving says.

It can take a heavy toll. A Stanford University study finds 40 percent of Alzheimer's and dementia caregivers die from stress-related disorders before the one for whom they are caring passes away. Sheria

Robinson-Lane, an assistant professor at the University of Michigan's School of Nursing, says researchers have found higher use of alcohol among caregivers, particularly those who are just beginning to care for a loved one with dementia.

But it's the increasing numbers of millennials and Gen Zers putting their own young lives on hold to help care for aging relatives that's especially startling to policymakers.

Susan Reinhard, director of AARP's Public Policy Institute, says she's met so many young caregivers who've ended up putting their own lives and studies on hold, "I started calling it 'Life Interrupted.'"

"One of them was a student who was trying to do homework at the hospital and sleeping on the floor. They're asking questions like, 'How do I explain the gap in my résumé?' 'How do I afford to rent an apartment when I have to spend so much on my parents?'" Reinhard says. Others feel like they can't confide in their peers about the toll it's taking on them: "They don't understand this. This isn't what they want to talk about at a party."

Schall, of the Caregiver Action Network, says many of these young caregivers are performing sophisticated acts that a doctor or a nurse traditionally would handle, such as administering medicine. He thinks high schoolers should be trained in how to provide basic care, much as earlier generations were taught home economics. "We need to put it really, really early in the life cycle," he says.

All of us, regardless of our stations in life, can find ourselves immersed in a caregiving situation. Even a Hollywood A-lister like Bradley Cooper.

The *A Star Is Born* actor and director took care of his father when he was terminally ill with cancer, and he acted as caregiver for his ailing octogenarian mother during the coronavirus pandemic and beyond. Cooper had moved in with his parents before his father's death in 2011. He drew from that painfully personal experience as executive producer of the 2023 PBS documentary *Caregiving*, says

Paul Irving, the Center for the Future of Aging founder we met first in chapter 5 and again in chapter 8.

"He recognized, 'Here I am. I'm this big Hollywood movie star, obviously with lots of resources and connections and all the rest, and it's incredibly difficult being a caregiver even under those circumstances. So, how must it be for people who are more challenged?'" says Irving, who worked with Cooper on the series.

In an emotional interview, Cooper opened up to Oprah Winfrey about the life-transforming moment of holding his father in his arms as he took his last breath:

> It was everything. It was the biggest gift he gave me—the second biggest gift: having me and bringing me into this life, and him allowing me to be witness to his passing was equally as huge. It really honestly felt like—he was cradled, his head was right here—and when he took the last breath, I honestly felt like it went into me. And I've never seen anything the same since.
>
> I stopped sweating stuff that I was sweating before that. It changed the way I was as an actor by, like, the next day, and I just started to live my life in a different way. I remember that moment and I looked up and I thought everything was different: stronger, more open, more willing to fail because of him. . . . The reality of mortality hits you like a ton of bricks.
>
> I love when he's in my dreams. In the beginning he was very sick in my dreams, and now in my dreams he's healthy.

Greg Link can relate. As director of the federal Administration for Community Living's Office of Supportive and Caregiver Services, he's been drawing up a national strategy aimed at ensuring caregivers can access the thorny patchwork of services available to them. It's work he's done for thirty-five years, but a decade ago, it took on a harrowing personal dimension—one Link rarely discusses because it's still so raw.

A New Yorker now, he was living in Washington, DC, when his aging parents in Fort Myers, Florida, began a slow descent into dementia. His mother was first; his father did everything he could for his wife of sixty-something years, but her health declined to the point that she needed nursing home care. Then his father began to suffer from dementia.

"I'll be very honest with you: There were days when I would be sitting out on the front porch sobbing, because I didn't know what to do," Link says. "I can help anybody else, but this became so personal. It has shaped everything that I do. You carry those caregiving scars with you. I'll never be the same. But I learned a lot. I have perspective. And I have no regrets of what I did and how I supported them. I never think back and say, 'I could have done more; I wish I'd done this.' I don't ask those questions."

Link's employer let him work remotely from Florida one week every month so he could support his father, monitor his care, and accompany him to medical appointments, and that flexibility was key.

That's another thing America needs to change: baking workplace flexibility into the culture so we can all more easily care for one another.

The exponential increase in remote work that began during the COVID-19 pandemic has given some caregivers a little more wiggle room. But only about a third of all workers can do their jobs remotely, notes Joseph Fuller, who codirects Harvard Business School's Project on Managing the Future of Work. Companies are slowly realizing there's a cost to staff turnover and an extra incentive to accommodate workers who need to care for their elders, Fuller says, much as they offer paid parental leave. "At different stages of life, people need different things from their employers," he says.

America's workforce participation rate has been tumbling for men and women since the early 2000s, and Fuller says caregiving responsibilities play a role in that decline. "It's now lower than virtually all of our peer competitors in the world," he says. "It's very often a punch line for Americans—'No one really works in France'—but France has a higher workforce participation rate than we do. That wasn't the case twenty-five years ago." Companies, he says, need to innovate and offer employees of all ages more flexibility so they can handle the complications thrown at them in every season of life.

Jennifer Wolff, a health policy researcher at Johns Hopkins University, says it's not as clear to companies when exactly an employee becomes a senior caregiver as it is when someone takes a break to care for a new child. In that scenario, you or your partner has a due date and a good sense of a return-to-work date. With an aging relative, Wolff concedes, "It can be a slow process: You start with some things here and there, some chores, and then suddenly you find yourself a few years later taking on increasingly more. How do employers decide which benefits are available and how to best allocate those benefits? At what point do you qualify for benefits? Those are much trickier questions."

Ruth Finkelstein, executive director of the Brookdale Center for Healthy Aging at New York City's Hunter College (whom we first met in chapter 5), thinks employers need to do more than pay lip service to the notion that "our workers are our greatest assets." If they really believe that, she insists, rather than dictating work hours, they should invoke something she calls "radical flexibility" by asking: "When is it good for you to work?" And conversely: "When is it impossible for you to work?"

. . .

THERE'S ANOTHER KIND OF CAREGIVER—PROFESSIONALS—AND they've probably got one of the toughest and most thankless jobs on Earth.

David Grabowski, a professor of health care policy at Harvard Medical School, says many professional caregivers in the United States are paid at or near the federal minimum, which isn't a living wage, and their earnings have stagnated for years.

There are 4.7 million professional direct care workers in the United States, helping provide care in private homes, assisted living facilities, nursing homes, and even prisons. (Talk about a hidden cost: By 2030, the number of elderly inmates in American prisons is expected to hit 400,000—a staggering 4,400 percent increase since 1981—with most destined to need expensive geriatric care.)

Most direct caregivers work wildly irregular hours; four in ten subsist at or below the poverty line; and the turnover rate is huge, meaning many seniors won't have continuity in terms of who's caring for them. Training requirements also vary widely from state to state. "So, as a family caregiver, if you hire a worker, you cannot be assured that they necessarily have trained and are equipped with the right skills or knowledge to succeed in their roles," says Robert Espinoza, executive vice president for policy at PHI, a national organization trying to strengthen the direct care profession.

During the COVID-19 pandemic, professional caregivers were deemed essential workers, but we didn't pay them or treat them as such. "In reality, their jobs are not valued as essential," Espinoza says. Yet between now and 2029, the long-term care sector will need to fill about 7.4 million job openings in direct care. University of California San Francisco researchers who looked at where vacancies were the highest found they're in the same region of the United States that has the most seniors with conditions that make them incapable of caring for themselves: the American South.

In my home state, the shortage of frontline caregivers is at a historic high. Workforce surveys conducted by the Massachusetts Senior Care Association show thousands of nurse vacancies—staffing shortages so acute that more than 60 percent of the state's nursing facilities are limiting admissions. Complicating that are hundreds of vacancies for housekeepers, dietary aides, cooks, activities assistants, and others. And that's despite supplemental government funding that helped those facilities raise wages by nearly 20 percent. Tara Gregorio, the organization's president, calls it "a persistent and alarming challenge."

Chronic understaffing at nursing homes and assisted living facilities has been a problem for decades. But as the sheer numbers of the elderly soar, it's going to get worse. A *USA Today* investigation finds that federal regulators have allowed thousands of nursing homes to go for twenty-four hours at a time without a single registered nurse on duty. Government inspectors cited only 4 percent of the offenders, and even fewer were fined, the investigation discovered, concluding: "When facilities are short-staffed, essential medical tasks are ignored. Doctor's appointments are missed, call buttons go unanswered, diapers are not changed, showers are not given, and wounds are not cleaned. Dementia can set in faster. People get sicker, and die alone."

Meanwhile, the US Department of Health and Human Services' Office of the Inspector General says eight in ten nursing home residents on Medicare are prescribed "chemical straitjacket" drugs—a class of psychiatric medications used to sedate unruly patients, especially those with dementia. AARP warns that their use all too often is "inappropriate and dangerous."

Little wonder that, like 108-year-old Juliet Bernstein, most of us vastly prefer to age in place, in our own homes, and arrange for whatever care we might need to come to us. That, however, is much more complicated than it sounds.

Some housing stock is in seriously rough shape; not easy for seniors to stay in. "We need a lot more residential options," says Robyn Stone, senior vice president for research at the University of Massachusetts Boston's LeadingAge Center. "Not everyone can stay in their own home." Rising rents and soaring inflation, meanwhile, are pushing a record number of seniors into the streets. Advocates project the number of low-income people aged fifty and older sliding into homelessness will nearly triple over the next decade, and they're going to need care that, like their rent, they can't afford.

And more boomers and Gen Xers than ever before are living alone. Riding the same demographic wave that's going to noticeably boost the number of centenarians among us, Americans aged fifty and up who live by themselves are one of the nation's fastest-growing segments of the population. Nearly 26 million fit that description, the US Census Bureau says. They're also far more likely to be unmarried, separated, or divorced, and to live far from their kids (if they've got any; about 15 percent don't have any children to look after them when they're older). Although many live full, healthy, contented, and remarkably active lives, their solitude doesn't set them up well for aging in place.

"The growth of solo living has important implications for the rising 'loneliness epidemic' among older adults," Baylor University sociologist Markus Shafer concludes in a new study examining the health implications of the go-it-alone lifestyle. "High levels of social connectedness only moderately buffer the loneliness associated with living alone in later life."

One solution is the Village Movement, an initiative launched two decades ago in Boston to connect people who are approaching retirement so they can help one another age in place. It's now a fixture in nearly every state, growing not only with the steady addition of boomers but of Gen Xers aware that retirement isn't so very distant for them, either. Members of these virtual villages grocery shop for one another, assist with doctor appointments and household services, and even help with the care and feeding of pets. Organizers say their goals are "reduced isolation, increased independence, and enhanced purpose of life."

Another is "age tech," an array of innovations being developed to help people stay in their homes as long as possible. A Dutch company, iZi (rhymes with "easy"), outfits seniors with hip-mounted airbags that deploy when they sense wearers are losing their balance so they don't break a hip. MIT's AgeLab is rewiring houses into "smart homes" with motion detectors that can alert emergency medical personnel to a fall; AI voice reminders to take medications; video links that let family members and others check in on the resident; and social robots like Miroki to perform basic tasks and keep them company.

Japan, the nation with the world's largest percentage of people aged sixty-five and older, has been rolling out robots as senior companions for nearly a decade, and the Japanese are welcoming them into their homes and assisted living facilities. The country represents where the United States is headed: a place where there are many more old citizens than young; where the number of elders vastly outstrips the ranks of caregivers; and where confidence in technology and artificial intelligence, misguided or not, is growing. One popular model sold by Fujisoft for roughly the equivalent of $6,000 is Palro, a compact dancing and singing humanoid "carebot" designed to help users combat dementia by taking them through fitness routines and trivia games.

Those are fine as far as they go, but as we age, two in three of us are going to need someone (read: a human) to help bathe us, dress us, and hoist us on and off the toilet. One glaringly obvious solution that's become equally problematic in Europe, Japan, and the United States: immigration. Employing more immigrants would help ease the caregiver shortage, provide jobs to newcomers who desperately need one, and prolong the time until we'll have to answer to our future robot overlords.

Win, win, win. Or it would be if our dysfunctional family of nations could somehow overcome our racist and xenophobic tendencies and take a more pragmatic approach to needlessly restrictive immigration policies.

One country that gets it is Canada, which has pledged to bring in nearly a million and a half immigrants by 2025 to fill critical jobs amid a persistent labor shortage.

Like so many other nations, Canada has an aging population and a lower birth rate. Immigrants are the country's best—some say only—bet to ensure its economy expands rather than shrinks. And Canada is more of a melting pot than the United States: One in four Canadians arrived as an immigrant, compared to one in seven Americans.

Whether Canada succeeds in its ambitious plan to fill caregiving vacancies and other jobs with immigrants remains to be seen. But hopes are high. "There is a degree of public trust that immigration to Canada is well-managed by the government and also is managed in a way that serves Canada's interests," Geoffrey Cameron, a political scientist at Ontario's McMaster University, tells the BBC.

EVERYONE LOVES A HERO—ESPECIALLY THE UNLIKELY VARIETY.

Meet Vida Bampoe, a remarkable immigrant caregiver who saved the day in the kind of nightmare scenario that could befall any of us in our centenarian future: an eighty-two-year-old woman looking after her 102-year-old mother.

The octogenarian is Mary Ann Evan, an IT specialist who spent the last part of her career working to protect Washington, DC's power grid from cyberterrorists. The centenarian: her mother, Angela, who'd moved in with her fifteen years earlier, initially living independently until she began suffering a series of falls. A bad one put her in the hospital, but she was prematurely discharged, and Mary Ann realized she wasn't strong enough to fully assist her, even though she'd had her single-level home retrofitted with a walk-in shower and bathroom grab bars.

"I was totally lost. I was just helpless," Mary Ann tells me. "It was clear to me that I needed a lot of help."

Enter Vida, a fifty-nine-year-old West Africa–born registered nurse. During the day, she coordinates resident care at a senior living center in DC, and at night, she moonlights as a privately paid home health aide.

"When I got to Mary Ann's [a client], her mom had been in a chair for probably two days," she recalls. "Before I went to work, I got her out of the chair, put her in bed, and made sure she was clean; and I showed up again in the evening. That was the routine for some time, until we switched to a twenty-four-hour rotation."

Presciently, Mary Ann's mother had arranged to advance her children their modest inheritance, and they spent $75,000 of it on her care. Two months later, she slipped away peacefully at home, in her own bed, where she'd always wanted to die. "The connection with Vida was a lifesaver," Mary Anne says, adding that because of her mother's experience, she's already starting to map out her own long-term care.

Vida, who immigrated to the United States from Ghana, imported one of her homeland's most cherished cultural values: providing loving and respectful care to elders. "My mom lived with me for twenty years, and what my children got out of that was: 'Do you need anything? Grandma, let me know if you need something,'" she says. "It's a cultural thing. We like to help in making a difference in the elder space." She's just one of tens of thousands of other immigrants who are poignantly and professionally filling America's caregiving niche.

But caregiving won't be our only worry if we live to 100. Making ends meet for a century or longer will be a particular challenge.

TWO WORDS STRIKE FEAR IN ALL BUT THE VERY WEALTHIEST OF US as we contemplate 100-year lives: *elder poverty*.

None of us wants to outlive our money, yet too many already are. One in ten Americans aged sixty-five and up is living in poverty, the National Council on Aging reports. More than half rely solely on Social Security, and even though they received a nearly 9 percent cost of living adjustment in 2023, the median monthly check of $1,778 is nowhere enough to keep pace with inflation and the skyrocketing cost of housing. (Nationally, rents went up 11 percent in 2022 on average, but more than three times that in many US cities.)

Over the next decade, the federal government will spend more than two-thirds of its budget on those aged sixty-five and older, mostly for Social Security and Medicare, the Congressional Budget Office projects. It forecasts the US government spending a staggering $3.4 trillion in 2029, a reflection of the population's dramatic aging.

It's no secret that Social Security needs urgent attention. The trust fund reserves underpinning the program are projected to run out of money just a decade from now. No one expects Congress to let the program implode—that's a political third rail—but if it doesn't act decisively by 2033, everyone on Social Security will get a 23 percent pay cut overnight: for many, an utterly unsurvivable blow. "There would be riots in the streets," says AARP's Whitman.

It's unlikely to come to that. Federal lawmakers can avert disaster through some combination of raising payroll taxes, reducing benefits, and once again upping the age at which we're eligible to start collecting full benefits. Sixty-five for decades, the full retirement age is now sixty-six years and four months for my wife; sixty-seven for me; and seventy for some of our slightly younger contemporaries.

A divided Congress is taking a hard look at making it seventy for everyone—an uphill battle that some lawmakers are already girding for, including Republican senator Susan Collins of Maine, who denounces withholding benefits until seventy as "regressive and unfair." Such moves are understandably unpopular. Consider France, where massive and violent protests erupted early in 2023 after President Emmanuel Macron bypassed parliament to push through a pension bill raising his country's retirement age from sixty-two to sixty-four. Bottom line: If there's ever been a convincing and publicly popular case to raise taxes on the wealthy, this is it.

Social Security has taken on an outsized role in the US retirement savings system simply because so few have either the discipline or the wherewithal to put anything aside. Bureau of Labor Statistics ex-commissioner William Beach says the median savings for retirement is just $30,000, which is woefully insufficient.

Half of the private sector workforce—an estimated 57 million people—don't have a retirement savings plan powered by automatic payroll deductions. Those who do find it difficult to migrate their 401(k) accounts from one employer to the next, and that means many people, especially those who earn less and people of color, end up cashing out their retirement savings when they leave a job. Life's relentless challenges—a flat tire, a leaky roof, a broken leg—often prompt people to spend that money rather than roll it into a new plan. "The people who need this the most to supplement their Social Security benefits are the ones who have it the least," says David John, a senior fellow in economic studies at the Brookings Institution think tank.

He advocates a more innovative system like the one in place in Australia, where retirement accounts follow workers from job to job throughout their working lives. "That way you don't lose any money. It just goes with you. And it continues to build up the way it should." The United Kingdom has been experimenting with a similar approach, John says, and it's seen significant increases both in the numbers of people saving for retirement and the amount of money they're setting aside.

Here's another bad habit that's eroding Americans' financial security in retirement: Too many of us start drawing our Social Security benefits too early; some when eligibility begins at age sixty-two, but for significantly lower amounts than if they'd wait for their full retirement age or later to get the maximum payout. Plus Social Security allowances are one of the few things indexed to inflation, so it's in everyone's best interest not to start drawing them too early at sharply reduced levels.

"As we plan for the 100-year life, the standard retirement playbook must evolve," says Lorna Sabbia, managing director of retirement and personal wealth solutions at Bank of America. She's part of a new, more holistic "financial wellness" movement that's encouraging us to focus beyond our retirement accounts and establish healthy rhythms of spending and saving, as well as thinking and preparing much earlier for the medical bills and other caregiving costs we'll all incur later in our lengthening lives. Making a wrong turn here, Sabbia warns, could be crippling.

In theory, working longer is an option—especially if more of us are going to see 100—but in practice, it's not so simple.

"The economic contribution of people over the age of fifty is real," says Jean Accius, AARP's vice president of global thought leadership. That's unquestionably true: In fact, the fastest-growing segment of the US population in terms of workforce participation is the seventy and older set. But there's a lot of inequity there. For every seventy-year-old with enough assets to start a business, a dozen are working as Walmart greeters or tending the fryers at McDonald's because they need the money.

"Why is it that working longer is not really a thing? Why is it that people cannot earn more now that they're living longer to supplement their Social Security and their retirement income? It's because jobs for older workers are not really what we typically think of. They're difficult jobs. They're physically demanding jobs," says Siavash Radpour of the New School for Social Research.

How long should we be expected to work? If we're going to live to 100, is it reasonable to think a lot of us are still going to be on the job in our eighties? Or is that just absurd?

"I don't see it myself," says Beth Truesdale, the W.E. Upjohn Institute sociologist we caught up with earlier. "Policies that rely on working longer, delaying retirement as the sort of core of how we respond to population aging, are likely to increase economic disparities because it's the people who've already had the best careers, the best health, the best education, the most money, who are most likely to be able to continue to work longer. Many, many people are not in that situation. I think we overlook how working longer is just not a workable proposition for so many."

That's especially true in the United States, Truesdale says. Nations like Germany and the Netherlands offer employees a greater voice to negotiate for policies that are responsive to the needs of older workers, helping them ease into retirement with greater financial security or shift into part-time work in the twilight of their careers. When they eventually need long-term care, they're treated with compassion, not warehoused. And it doesn't bankrupt them. In fact, they're still able to leave money and property to their children, preserving the kind of generational wealth that helps their kids buy a home—an inheritance windfall that's going to vanish for future generations of Americans.

"People should have leisure and they should be able to do whatever they like with those years at the end of a long working career," she adds. "I think there's something very attractive about that as a proposition. I don't think we should, as a society, think our goal is to get everybody to work as long as they possibly can, or to wring every last ounce of productivity out of every last person."

That leaves governments and ordinary citizens to pick up the tab for seniors' care. And with the costs so astronomically high, it can have geopolitical consequences.

China's population is aging so rapidly and profoundly that it's going to have to spend enormous sums on pensions and health care. An illuminating analysis by the RAND Corporation global think tank concludes that as the Chinese government spends more on social programs, "these demands will limit the resources China has available for military spending." By 2025, Chinese people are expected to account for a quarter of the world's sixty-plus population.

Beijing is taking those changing demographics and the need to ensure seniors receive adequate care seriously—a little too seriously, perhaps, by Western standards: There's an elder rights law on the books that exposes children to potential prison time, fines, and public shaming if they don't support their aging parents and visit them regularly. It's all part of a deeply held virtue in Chinese society that's known as filial piety: a 2,500-year-old cultural expectation that dates to Confucius and demands that elders are respected and revered.

It's interesting that even in a communist country like China, there's pressure to make sure seniors have the resources and care they need.

In the United States, you can purchase private long-term care insurance, but fewer than 7 percent of Americans have a policy. It's not cheap: Coverage for a fifty-five-year-old couple runs about $5,000 a year. And with Medicare not covering long-term nursing care, our fates can come down to the kindness of strangers.

In a high-profile and moving case that stirred hearts and grabbed headlines a few years ago, singer/songwriter and Hollywood actor Chris Salvatore, then thirty-one, invited his childless eighty-nine-year-old neighbor, Norma Cook, to live with him so he could care for her as her death from leukemia approached. The *Catfish Killer* star also raised more than $77,000 for Cook's medical expenses.

When she died the day after Valentine's Day, Salvatore posted on Instagram:

Norma has helped the world see the true meaning of Valentine's Day. To love another is not about living struggle free or never experiencing hurt or loss, but to fully and deeply open our hearts to one another without fear. Each of us is lovable even with all of our differences. Love has no boundaries.

LOVE, IT TURNS OUT, IS LINKED TO LONGEVITY.

Born on the Fourth of July, 108-year-old Izer Tilson of Rockford, Illinois, married his high school sweetheart, and they raised fifteen children who gave him more than 100 grandchildren.

Experts say belief and positivity are keys to an exceptionally long life—something we'll explore in the next chapter. Determination and a sense of humor don't hurt, either. As the iconic entertainer Dick van Dyke, who's closing in on 100, likes to crack:

In my thirties, I exercised to look good; in my fifties, to stay fit; in my seventies, to stay ambulatory; in my eighties, to avoid assisted living. Now, in my nineties, I'm just doing it out of pure defiance.

CHAPTER TEN

BELIEF, POSITIVITY, AND THE TRUTH ABOUT "BLUE ZONES"

I'm generally a glass-half-full kind of guy. I like my eggs sunny side up. Even my blood type is B-positive.

You get the picture. And scientists say I have even more to be optimistic about: They've established a clear correlation between positivity and longevity. Researchers say people who embrace a religious faith (I do), and others who care more for the common good than for their individual wellness (I'm working on it), stand a markedly better chance of achieving a triple-digit age.

Even so, my hopefulness could never hold a candle to the optimism my father-in-law radiated against all odds and reason.

Though he'd endured a decades-long and relentless physical decline that required him to use a cane, a walker, and eventually a motorized cart, Gene DeYonker lived a long, full, and improbably happy life. *"Never been better"* was his mantra right up to his death, and he invoked it often—occasionally under hilarious circumstances.

Once on a whim, while my wife and I were living in Europe, I phoned Gene at his home in the Detroit suburbs just to hear how he was doing. He picked up with characteristic good cheer, and we made small talk before he mentioned in passing that he hoped my mother-in-law would be returning soon from the grocery store:

"Why's that, Dad?" I asked.
"Oh, nothing. It's just that I flipped my cart over and I've been lying here on the ground for the last hour and a half."
"Whaaaaaaaaaaaaaaat?! Are you okay?!"
"Never been better. I've got a cold beer that only spilled a little, and the grass is nice and soft, and it's a beautiful day to be outside."

Now *that's* positivity. Little wonder he'd live to eighty-one; a good seven years longer than average life expectancy for someone with multiple sclerosis.

You don't get to 122 years and 164 days without a little irreverence and a lot of humor.

Jeanne Calment's life was the longest ever, though certainly not the easiest. To be sure, she enjoyed more than a dozen decades of white privilege and affluence along with her jackpot of favorable genes. But she was no stranger to heartache. Her only daughter died at age thirty-six of pneumonia, and her husband's life was cut tragically short when he was poisoned by a dessert of spoiled cherries at age forty-six, leaving her a widow for more than half a century. She comforted herself after her daughter's death by raising her grandson, but he, too, died young in a car crash.

French longevity researcher Jean-Marie Robine, who spent hundreds of hours in Calment's company, believes her virtual immunity to stress played a key role in her staying power. And the grand dame herself credited laughter for her life span. Both come through in some of her more memorable witticisms:

"Always keep your smile. That's how I explain my long life."
"Every age has its happiness and troubles."
"I think I will die laughing."
"I never wear mascara . . . too often I laugh until I cry."

"Always look on the bright side of life," Eric Idle sang as he was being crucified in Monty Python's *Life of Brian*, and he was on to something. Researchers at Boston University's School of Medicine, examining how optimism affects our health by following 233 older men over a period of fourteen years, found it appears to promote emotional well-being by helping us handle daily stress more con- structively. Although the underlying mechanisms at play remain

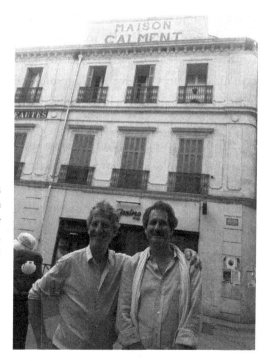

Renowned gerontologists Tom Perls and Jean-Marie Robine outside the Calment family department store in Arles, France (*Leslie Smoot*)

unclear: "By looking at whether optimistic people handle day-to-day stressors differently, our findings add to knowledge about how optimism may promote good health as people age," says Lewina O. Lee, a clinical psychologist who coauthored the study.

Lee also participated in a separate study of a racially and socio-economically diverse group of nearly 160,000 women aged fifty to seventy-nine in the United States. It found those who scored highest on evaluations of optimism levels were 10 percent more likely to live beyond ninety. "Higher optimism was associated with longer life span and a greater likelihood of achieving exceptional longevity overall," the researchers conclude.

And for those of us who, like me, have had it with the rat race, scientists at Penn State University have some heartening news: The amount of daily stress we experience as we age tends to decrease, and so does our reactivity to it, which is where things can get toxic for us.

That team collected copious data from the daily lives of more than 3,000 people over two decades, and they interviewed the subjects periodically to check in on their stress levels. The twenty-five-year-olds in the study said they felt stressed nearly half of the time; the seventy-year-olds were stressed out 30 percent of the time. That's still a lot of grief and hassle, but at least the trend lines are comforting.

In an enlightening study of how Americans perceive the second half of their lives compared to the first half, AARP and National Geographic surveyed 2,580 adults aged eighteen and older, and about two in three of the oldest—those aged eighty and above—said they were living their best lives. Only one in five of the youngest respondents could say the same. "While people recognize some of the challenges that come with aging, many have an optimistic outlook and expect their lives to improve as they grow older," the researchers say.

It helps to become exceptionally old in a city. Nearly nine in ten centenarians live in urban centers, which typically provide public transit options, readier access to health care services, greater opportunities to connect socially with others, and more cultural and sports activities. And at any age, but especially 100, staying in touch with dear ones is key: About the same percentage say they communicate with a relative or friend almost every day.

TimeSlips founder Anne Basting, whom we met in chapter 6, sees more brightness than bleakness as we age.

"There is happiness and sadness in young people's and middle-aged people's lives. We have both. But somehow we only see the tragedy and the loss in the last part of life. I'm just repairing that to a balance, you know, because of course there's beauty in every day. You're alive, for God's sake, even if it's bleak," she tells me.

"I think about *Life Is Beautiful*, the Roberto Benigni film about the Holocaust, where the guy decides he's going to play with his kid through the concentration camp because you can't pull play and meaning out of life entirely or you're not alive. There is happy and sad, and we have to have both in our lives—all the way to the end."

The French have a perfect expression for this: *Être bien dans sa peau*—to feel good in one's skin. It's positive self-affirmation, even if our circumstances are less than ideal. As we age, anything we can do to shed stress and put ourselves in a happy place emotionally is worthwhile, if only because the alternative is unacceptable. US Centers for Disease Control and Prevention figures bear tragic witness to that: Among older adults, drug and alcohol deaths are on the rise, including a staggering 53 percent increase in fatal overdoses from fentanyl and other synthetic opioids by people aged sixty-five and up.

More than mere wishful thinking, positive beliefs around aging have the potential to extend our lives by as much as seven-and-a-half years, according to research by Becca Levy, an epidemiologist at Yale University's School of Public Health. The cumulative effects of an optimistic outlook even outweigh the steps we take to exercise, lower our blood pressure and cholesterol, and watch our weight—possibly because those who take a sanguine approach to life are twice as likely as pessimists to do all those things as well as eat healthy, refrain from smoking, and go easy on the booze. Perhaps not coincidentally, cheery seniors enjoy more friendships, visits, and offers of help than grouchy ones, not just extending life but enhancing its meaning and quality.

"The way in which individuals view their own aging affects their functional health," Levy's team concludes. "Those with more positive self-perceptions of aging . . . have better functional health over time than those with more negative self-perceptions." And a lot of that is obviously up to us: As we age, we have a bothersome tendency to think of ourselves as old.

What is old, anyway? wonders Madeline Smith, a youthful ninety-nine. Smith, who still plays tennis with her younger contemporaries in Connecticut, says she's deeply grateful to have been spared much of the tragedy and tribulation that can roil our lives. "A lot of it is the attitude," she tells the *Republican American* newspaper. "I've had a few ups and downs, but it doesn't really hang on to me. I try to always see the positive and not focus on the negative. I think I'm going to live another ten years at least."

Life can get heavy, so keeping things light and having a little cheeky fun whenever possible is always a good idea. When I turn 100, I'm stealing a page from centenarian Jean Bicketon's playbook. A life-long law abider, the Australian who served as an Army nurse during World War II celebrated her 100th birthday with a bucket-list experience: getting arrested. Local police were happy to oblige, arriving at her party with lights flashing and sirens blaring to handcuff her and lead her outside to a waiting patrol car.

As Madame Calment was fond of saying: "If you can't do anything about it, don't worry about it."

Author Anne Lamott puts it this way: "A hundred years from now? All new people." (She also says this: "Life has got to be bigger than death, and love has got to be bigger than fear, or this is all a total bust and we are all just going tourist class." But more on the life-extending power of love a little later.)

HAD YOU ASKED JUAN VICENTE PÉREZ MORA THE SECRET TO HIS longevity, the Venezuelan who was the world's oldest man when he died a month before his 115th birthday, likely would have answered as he always did: "Love God and always carry him in your heart." Pérez Mora, who prayed the rosary twice a day, said what he treasured most was "the love of God, the love of family."

Japan's Kane Tanaka, who died in 2022 as the world's then-oldest living person, voiced similar sentiments over her 119 years and 107 days. A convert to Christianity from Shinto, she frequently attributed her longevity to her faith.

Spirituality is the tie that binds many centenarians and super-centenarians. National Geographic and the Blue Zones organization interviewed 263 people aged 100 or older, and all but five belonged to a faith community. Subsequent research suggests attending religious services four times a month can add at least four years of extra life span. Researchers at Ohio State University found something similar after analyzing more than a thousand obituaries to see who listed a religious affiliation; those who did lived 5.64 years longer on average than those who didn't.

That squares with the findings of a much larger long-term study suggesting regularly attending religious services can increase life span. A team at the Harvard T.H. Chan School of Public Health examined data collected over a twenty-year period from nearly 75,000 middle-aged female US nurses who were free of cardiovascular disease and cancer when the study began. Regardless of race or ethnicity, those who attended a temple, synagogue, mosque, or church at least once a week had a 33 percent diminished risk of death from all causes—but especially heart attack, stroke, and cancer—compared to those who never went.

"Religion and spirituality may be an underappreciated resource that physicians could explore with their patients," the researchers say. The "whys" remain elusive, though some scientists think abstinence from drugs and alcohol—common to many faiths—may help explain the benefits, along with the stress-relieving power of prayer and meditation. There's also the sense of community and belonging, which can counter the life-sapping effects of loneliness and isolation we explored in chapter 6.

"Religion and spirituality play an important role in the lives of older adults, as they help older people find meaning in later life," concludes a team of Portuguese researchers who took a closer look at 121 centenarians and their will—or not—to live.

Anecdotally, you'll find plenty of exceptionally old people who attribute their longevity to their faith. And for many, the explanation is divine.

"I think faith comes first," says 105-year-old Julia Kopriva, asked by a reporter for her advice as she celebrated a birthday with her sisters, aged 100 and 102.

"The secret is the grace of God living in me and me trying to live the best life that I could," adds 100-year-old Martha Bailey.

"Cigars and God," quipped Richard Overton, who made it to 112 as America's oldest surviving World War II veteran, apparently hedging his bets.

Christianity has something interesting to say about extreme longevity that's long captured my imagination. Was the Old Testament prophet Isaiah peering into our future when he penned these lines?

Never again will there be an infant who lives but a few days, or
an old man who does not live out his years;

The one who dies at a hundred will be thought a mere child; the one who fails to reach a hundred will be considered accursed.

Indeed, all the major faith traditions offer a grab bag of hope and instruction around extended life span.

The Talmud promises it to Jews who live a righteous life based on ethics and morals. It tells of Benjamin the Righteous, who had twenty-two years added to his life because of his acts of charity, which saved the lives of a woman and her seven children suffering during a famine.

Islam's holy book, the Quran, directly addresses cognitive impairment—"Of you there are some who are sent back to a feeble age, so that they know nothing after having known (much)"—while suggesting Muslims can live to 100 if they show kindness and maintain good relations with their family.

Buddhism offers keys to health and longevity: Don't abuse or torment other living beings; show sympathy when we see them suffering; and never let our parents suffer deprivation.

Hinduism, too, teaches the importance of caring for aging elders: "No person can repay his parents even in 100 years for all the troubles that they go through to give birth to him and raise him to adulthood."

And the apostle Paul reminds us that the biblical admonition to honor our fathers and mothers is the first commandment with a promise: "Things will go well for you, and you will have a long life on the Earth."

We've looked at longevity through the lens of science, not faith, but some of our greatest scientific thinkers see no incompatibility between the two. Among them is Dr. Jane Goodall, who describes in chapter 1 her fascination with what happens to us when we die. She speaks with childlike wonder about experiencing God not only in

Notre-Dame cathedral but in the forests of Gombe, Tanzania, where she first studied chimpanzees in the wild. Both sorts of encounters, she says, have sustained and enlivened her over her nine decades and counting.

"I think more and more scientists are coming to terms" with faith, she tells me. "My mother never saw a conflict; nor did Louis Leakey. Einstein was a great proponent of that. Francis Collins, who's just retired as director of the National Institutes of Health, started off agnostic and his science caused him to rethink. What is the conflict, really, between believing in an intelligent power and believing in evolution and all the rest of it?" Then, elaborating:

> When I was in the forest, I had this very strong spiritual connection with the natural world and became more and more convinced of intelligence behind the universe, which is what some of the best scientific minds have concluded.
>
> It hit me for the first time when I was thirty-something, going through a rather bad patch. I was in Notre-Dame cathedral early in the morning on my own, and the sun was just coming through that great rose window, and suddenly an organ started up with Bach's Toccata and Fugue in G minor. Apparently a couple were having an early morning wedding. And it just came over me that this can't be chance. I was thinking of all the amazing brains that had created the cathedral, and all the sort of strange couplings that led to Bach, and I don't know, there I was. It was a very strange awakening.
>
> I had the same sort of feeling in the forest. I had this feeling, you know, that everything's interconnected. It was as though each living thing had a little spark of that great spiritual power. And because we call things names all the time, we use words, we call that a soul or a spirit. If I have a soul or a spirit, so does a chimp and so does a bee. It's just what we choose to call it.

I was very traditionally religious when I was an adolescent because my grandfather was a congregational minister. We went to church sometimes, not very often; we weren't a religious family at all. But, you know, the Bible was always around, and lots of quotations from the Bible. And then I fell platonically in love with a parson who was a Welshman with a beautiful voice. I went to every service I possibly could, and it was very real to me at that time—very real to me. But then, you know, I went out into the world and it sort of got forgotten. And then this spiritual thing came back in the forest. When you talk about faith with people being old, my grandmother had a great faith. Think of the shamans: They live to be very, very old, many of them, and they live ascetic lives.

Goodall, by the way, doesn't think much of contemporary religious conservatives who profess belief but reject science and embrace an exclusionary brand of nationalism.

"I'm afraid their belief in God is not the kind of belief that any God that I know would approve of," she says. "Every single major religion shares the same golden rule: Do to others as you would have them do to you. If everybody obeyed that rule, the world would be a wonderful place."

A prolific author, Goodall supercharges her books with two recurrent themes: hope and optimism. Are they the same thing? I ask. Not exactly, she says.

"A lot of optimism can be in the genes, it seems—you have an optimistic nature—but that can also be cultivated in the child. For me, hope is different. I'm optimistic everything's going to be all right. But hope? Yes, you want it to be all right. You see a goal. There's a dark tunnel, but at the end of it, there's a little gleam of light if we can only get there. And that's hope. We will only get there if we work, if we try, if we do our very best. Hope is determined by action. That's my definition."

Religion also is a factor in the blue zones, which we'll examine next. But fair warning: Read on before you pack up and buy a
farmhouse on Sardinia, a minka on Okinawa, or a villa on Ikaria,
because it turns out they're not quite the centenarian factories they
may seem.

IN THE 1990s, BELGIAN DEMOGRAPHER MICHEL POULAIN FIDDLED
with a blue ballpoint pen as he bent over a map of Sardinia, a rugged
Italian island in the Mediterranean.

A few locations intrigued him—especially the mountainside
municipality of Villagrande Strisaili, where he'd noticed three things
were plentiful: homemade ricotta, locally sourced extra virgin olive
oil, and centenarians. A disproportionately large number of villagers
seemed to live to 100, and Poulain wanted to know more. He circled
the town in blue ink, and the term "blue zone" was coined. Today,
longevity experts have identified four others: Costa Rica's Nicoya
Peninsula; the Greek island of Ikaria in the Aegean Sea; Okinawa,
Japan; and Loma Linda, California, the Seventh-day Adventist
enclave we visited in chapters 3 and 6.

They're still puzzling over the impressive life spans and health
spans of these places' inhabitants. Diet alone certainly doesn't
explain it. Indeed, while nearly all blue zone seniors consume red
meat sparingly, if at all, some eat a diet heavy in fish and light on
dairy, and others consume large amounts of milk and cheese. Far
more than nutrition is at play, complicating if not negating the bar-
rage of prescriptive and contradictory messages—"Don't eat this!
Definitely eat that!"—bombarding the rest of us.

From Dr. Tom Perls, our longevity expert, comes an inconvenient
truth: Although people live demonstrably longer and healthier in
blue zones—more enjoy their nineties with remarkable vibrancy—
they don't produce significantly more centenarians. As we've seen,

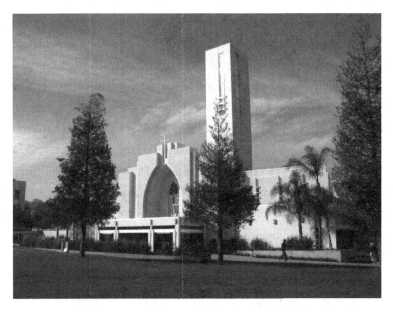

Loma Linda, California, is a center of the Seventh-day Adventist Church, whose members tend to live a decade longer than other Americans. (*© Jaime de la Fuente via Creative Commons*)

people who manage to reach 100 do so in a remarkably stable ratio of one in 5,000 virtually everywhere in the world.

Dr. Saul Newman, a researcher at Oxford University and Australian National University, more bluntly calls into question the data. Longevity records can be imprecise in the blue zones: Literacy rates are lower, with the exception of Loma Linda, and people have a tendency to fib about their age. In a 2019 analysis, Newman offers evidence to "support a primary role of fraud and error in generating remarkable human age records." And nutritionist David Lightsey challenges the notion of Okinawa as a Fountain of Youth, writing in a commentary for the American Council on Science and Health: "Outside of a small overall number of genetically prone individuals living to 100, the overall life expectancy for Okinawans is not significantly different."

Even so, there's a lot we can learn from blue zoners.

For starters, they tend not to be obese. They don't smoke. They stop eating when they're 80 percent full. They get their exercise and gain cardiovascular fitness not by running marathons like me, or by pumping iron in the gym, but by moving naturally through their environments as they work and walk from place to place. They get plenty of sleep. They maintain close family ties. And, perhaps most crucially, they enjoy these lifestyles largely free of stress.

"Chronic stress is a major pandemic of the developed countries in the twenty-first century and it is usually associated with work or money," notes a team of longevity scientists from the University of Nicosia in Cyprus. They've noticed something else common to all five blue zones that hasn't been closely examined: ecological concern and respect for the planet. "This might even contribute to their wellbeing and longevity," they say, urging more study. "Some of the possible explanations could be the reduced indoor and outdoor pollution, the presence of a balanced food chain and ecosystem, and healthy flora and fauna."

German demographer Marc Luy, curious why women in general outlive men by three or more years, is running a long-term study of 12,000 nuns and monks in Bavaria and neighboring Austria. What he's found suggests the gender gap in life expectancy may have more to do with lifestyle than biological differences. The nuns still live a year longer than the monks, but their shared way of life closes the gap—and both sexes in the monasteries outlive by five years their counterparts in the far more stressful workaday world.

Something particularly profound the blue zones share? They are "We Cultures" rather than "Me Cultures." Members of "We Cultures" care more for the community than for themselves, and they thrive in a small-town sense of being connected. That extends to how they care for their elders, who tend to live in family-focused, multigenerational pods. Far from being isolated, they enjoy a cradle-to-grave existence where the greatest common denominator is life-giving—gerontologists would say life-extending—interaction with others. That's in stark contrast to the physical and social isolation increasingly shrouding so many of us, especially in Western society, although that may be changing: The Pew Research Center says one in five Americans lived in a multigenerational home in 2021.

All of these blue zone virtues are being replicated in four dozen locations around North America as regional and municipal governments seek to enhance the well-being of their local populations.

Just one example: The Blue Zones organization is partnering with officials in California's Riverside County to identify what can be improved in neighborhoods, parks, and other places where residents spend the most time—things like modifying street designs, planting trees to shade and cool urban centers, and adding paths for walking and biking—to help them live healthier and longer.

Blue Zones is doing something similar in the city of Coachella, which hosts the eponymous annual music and arts festival, to see what aspects of the community can be tweaked to help people live closer to 100. Outside the United States, there's a project underway in Alberta, Canada, and more are planned. Organizers claim to have helped participating cities achieve "double-digit drops in obesity and smoking, millions of dollars of health care savings, and measurable drops in employee absenteeism."

There's something else linked to longevity that's harder to measure: a heartfelt reason to live.

You'll find in many centenarians an energizing and contagious sense of purpose.

DR. EPHRAIM ENGLEMAN, A 104-YEAR-OLD RHEUMATOLOGIST, DIED as he lived: at work, at his desk, in-between seeing patients at the

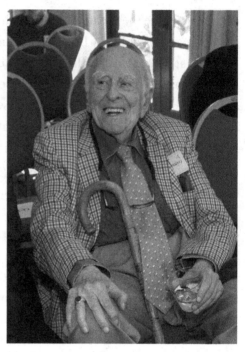

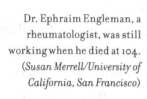

Dr. Ephraim Engleman, a
rheumatologist, was still
working when he died at 104.
(*Susan Merrell/University of
California, San Francisco*)

Rosalind Russell Medical Research Center for Arthritis in San
Francisco.

Engleman very deliberately never retired, a move he regarded
with suspicion as "generally a great mistake." One of his top rules
for longevity was: "Enjoy your work, whatever it is, or don't do it."

Robert Marchand, a diminutive Frenchman, was told he'd never
excel in cycling. Determined to prove his detractors wrong, he set
world records as a centenarian. He was still riding his exercise bike
twenty minutes a day not long before he died at 109.

Both men's drive, deep into their triple-digit life spans, underscores the importance of having something to live for. It's a characteristic common to many centenarians, and most of the time, their
resolve is evident long before that 100th birthday candle is lit.

Researchers in Portugal studied 121 centenarians to get a better
idea of whether life at 100 is worth living. Only a third indicated they

didn't want to live longer, and a common explanation beyond poor health was a lack of purpose in life. Those content to continue aging into their 100s, by contrast, found meaning and satisfaction in celebrating family achievements such as seeing a grandchild graduate from university or marry, or meeting a new great-grandchild. "Will to live is a strong predictor for survival among older people, irrespective of age, gender, and comorbidities," the team says.

Mimi Reinhard had it. A secretary in Oskar Schindler's office who typed up the list of 1,200 Jews he saved from extermination by Nazi Germany, she lived to 107. Her son, Sasha Weitman, says the Steven Spielberg blockbuster *Schindler's List*, which won a best picture Oscar, made her a celebrity and "pumped another fifteen years into her life."

Perls, who's met with hundreds of centenarians over the past few decades, says some of his most memorable encounters have been with those still energized by passions and interests they've cultivated since their youth.

Extreme sports like free climbing or skydiving aside, if we loved something in our twenties, who's to say we can't keep pursuing it in our 100s?

"One lady I remember: Celia," he told a Boston University podcast. "She was 102 and she was never around for me to go visit her at this independent living community. I thought maybe she was out seeing her doctors or something. But no, she was out playing piano at all kinds of gigs—really complex Chopin."

Daniela Jopp, a noted Swiss psychologist and aging expert leading a study of centenarians in Switzerland that's due to be completed in 2024, says she's noticed the same phenomenon: very old people still showing tremendous vitality, living lives of determination and intention.

"For example, a centenarian from the US whom I interviewed as part of a study regularly invited her friends and a Buddhist monk to meditate together. She was 101 or 102 at the time," Jopp tells the

Austrian newsmagazine *Profil*. "A 103-year-old man from a small town in western Switzerland was very refreshing. We wrote to him about a study. A day later he called and was keen to take part but was in a bit of a hurry because he was flying to New York in a few days to visit his great-granddaughter."

A beloved 1868 Currier & Ives lithograph, *The Four Seasons of Life: Old Age*, captures the contentment the twilight of our lives can offer. It depicts an elderly couple sitting by a crackling fireplace in the parlor of their home on a cold winter's day. He's reading a newspaper; she's knitting; and their granddaughter is reciting from a book in her lap. To the Michele and Donald D'Amour Museum of Fine Arts in Springfield, Massachusetts, the message is clear: "Although winter symbolizes life's final season, the pair quietly enjoy the knowledge that their grandchild represents the coming spring."

Mike Fremont, the 102-year-old runner we met in chapter 3, is taking a far more active approach to his eleventh decade. Fremont, who holds four age-group world records, also engages in climate activism. He tells fitness author and podcaster Rich Roll: "The conclusion I came to long, long ago was that the real satisfaction that people can get in their lifetimes consists in helping other people. Period. In whatever way, as much as you can. That brings real rewards."

That's the spirit, says Bill McKibben, the Th!rd Act founder we caught up with in chapter 8. More than 40,000 people from across the United States aged sixty and older—including several in their 100s—have joined the organization, eager to take to the streets to protect the climate and democracy.

"The key is this word 'legacy.' It's quite an abstract word," McKibben tells me. "But it becomes real when you have kids or grandkids or other people you care about. Your legacy is the world you leave behind for those you love the most, and the one we're leaving behind at the moment is on track to be shabbier than the one we inherited. We may be the first generation for which that's true. That's not the legacy that you want. We'll have to fight to make it different, and I think that's why people are locking in and doing it with real purpose."

McKibben, sixty-four, has stern words for anyone sporting his least-favorite bumper sticker: *I'm spending my kids' inheritance.*

"It's really not all that funny. It's really kind of gross," he says. "The problems we're having with the climate and democracy will have to be solved soon." And time is not on the side of senior activists: "We're closer to the exit than the entrance at this point."

LOVE CONQUERS ALL. EVEN DEATH—TO SOME EXTENT, ANYWAY.

Researchers say married people tend to live longer than singles— men by two-and-a-half years; women by a little less—and they also stand a better chance of living to 100, even though that can mean outliving the very partner whose security and affection helped get them there.

Tension and conflict in marriage are stand-up comedy staples, but studies have shown that those of us who endure the vicissitudes of life with a partner experience less stress than those who go solo. Couples have greater life expectancy free of disability and other health challenges than singles. And they tend to have more financial security, despite what my bemused father told me on the eve of my own wedding: "Remember, Bill, two can live as cheaply as one—for half as long."

There's also the obvious social benefit of marriage as an antidote to loneliness, at least in happy unions. (It's not an exact science: Researchers investigating the role of marriage in longevity acknowledge some built-in selection bias, since physically and mentally healthy people are more likely to marry in the first place.)

A wild card in all this is the stubbornly high divorce rate among baby boomers, who are driving the coming wave of centenarians. Despite a decline since 1980 in the overall US divorce rate, it's up among those over fifty, and over the past half century it has tripled among Americans aged sixty-five and older.

Nearly 40 percent of people who are sixty-five to seventy-four, and a quarter of those who are seventy-five and up, have dissolved a marriage, the US Census Bureau says. Sociologists and gerontologists call this phenomenon "gray divorce," and it's unclear what, if any, effect it will have as those who have consciously uncoupled approach old age alone. No two divorces are alike. Some enjoying newfound freedom from the toxic stress of a combative marriage may add to their life spans; others suddenly thrust into the strain of solitude may die before their time.

It's not the sex, the tax deductions, or even the cohabitation that make marriage so beneficial. Deep platonic friendships can have the same effect.

At an assisted living facility in Montana, two centenarians have found beauty and meaning in a relationship that's blossomed around their shared love of poetry. Bob Yaw is 101; Gloria Hansard is 100. They live down the hall from each other but gather each evening in her apartment to recite verses. "We didn't meet long ago," Hansard tells the *Bozeman Daily Chronicle*. "Just poems are all we know of each other."

Their friendship is life-giving and beautiful, with a soundtrack straight out of Frank Sinatra's "Young at Heart":

And if you should survive to 105
Look at all you'll derive
Out of being alive

·   ·   ·

I LIVE IN A 100-YEAR-OLD HOUSE THAT STANDS ON THE TRADI-tional homeland of the Narragansett Nation. Only about 2,400 members remain, but their tribe is one of North America's oldest, and they've been a presence here for 11,000 years. Just knowing I walk in their footsteps is, for me, big medicine.

That's another way to measure human longevity: not in terms of individual lives, but collectively, in the staying power of neighborhoods; communities; nations.

I've always been struck by the gentleness and humility of indigenous people. "Walk softly on the Earth," says Big Toe, a contemporary Narragansett elder here in Rhode Island. Lately, though, I've been ruminating on a truth voiced a century and a half ago by a tribal leader on the other side of the vast landmass known to some native people in their common and colorful creation story as Turtle Island and to the rest of us as North America.

"Humankind has not woven the web of life. We are but one thread within it," sagely observed the Duwamish tribe's Chief Si'ahl, namesake of the city of Seattle, in the early 1800s. "Whatever we do to the web, we do to ourselves. All things are bound together. All things connect."

With the Webb space telescope, suddenly we're able to peer into Sagittarius A, the supermassive black hole 26,000 light-years away in the center of the Milky Way. NASA calls it our Galileo moment. What we really need, though, is a universal epiphany down here on Earth.

Much within these pages isn't debatable. It's destiny. Boomers are aging in numbers massive enough to octuple (that's right, multiply by eight) the ranks of centenarians within a few short decades, and life-extending medical breakthroughs are occurring both at a breathtaking pace and an unprecedented scale. Those are facts, and they're going to significantly lengthen our lives. Unfortunately, these are also facts: Not everyone on the planet will benefit, and the humanity that Chief Si'ahl insists connects us all also demands that we care. In the spirit of Carl Sagan: "Every one of us is, in the cosmic perspective, precious."

As a foreign correspondent, I spent weeks at a time on assignment in the lush and lively West African nation of Côte d'Ivoire, and I came to treasure the Ivorians' warmth and the richness of their culture. Ornate tribal masks elegantly carved from albizia hardwood decorate our home. A recurrent theme is the *tête de beliye*, or ram's head, an ancient symbol of strength, stability, and longevity. But those things—especially longevity—are in short supply in Côte d'Ivoire.

Average life expectancy there is just 60.3 years, plunging the country nearly to the bottom of the World Health Organization's global rankings. In fact, the ten nations with the lowest life expectancies are all in Africa—Central African Republic, Chad, Lesotho, Nigeria, Sierra Leone, Somalia, Côte d'Ivoire, South Sudan, Guinea Bissau, and Equatorial Guinea—and they're also among those most vulnerable to climate catastrophes such as famine. Bloodied by deadly intercommunal fighting, the mineral-rich but impoverished Nigeria is rock bottom at 54.1 years. Some of us may wind up living twice as long as that.

"All babies are beautiful," 122-year-old Jeanne Calment declared. Many infants in Africa, however, live to a ripe old age far less frequently. Yet that barely registers on a binary planet divided between the developed and the developing; the haves and the have-nots; the long- and the short-lived. It spins on, oblivious to what we've been given and they've been denied: twenty-five more years of everything, including love, laughter, and dreams.

Meanwhile, not content with all of that, we grab greedily at life with both hands, popping dubious supplements and obsessing over the latest fad diets in a compulsive attempt to cheat death. Ezekiel Emanuel, a University of Pennsylvania bioethicist whose incisive essay in *The Atlantic*, "Why I Hope to Die at 75," touched off a spirited national debate, ridicules what he calls the culture of the American immortal. But he gets why we do it:

"After all, evolution has inculcated in us a drive to live as long as possible. We are programmed to struggle to survive. Consequently, most people feel there is something vaguely wrong with saying seventy-five and no more. We are eternally optimistic Americans who chafe at limits, especially limits imposed on our own lives. We are sure we are exceptional."

(We're not, incidentally: US life expectancy in 2024 was ranked fifty-eighth, just below Lebanon and just ahead of the Falkland Islands. In case you're curious, the ten countries where people live the longest, in descending order, are Monaco, Hong Kong, Macau, Japan, Liechtenstein, Switzerland, Singapore, Italy, South Korea, and Spain.)

What's an extra year of good health worth to you? The average American would pay $242,000 for a hypothetical intervention that accomplished that, according to an analysis by Andrew Scott, a professor of economics at London Business School. It's only a matter of time before Big Pharma develops a cost-prohibitive class of drugs capable of slowing or reversing the aging process and postponing death. Society—that's us—will have to decide whether anyone who isn't wealthy gets access.

"Undoubtedly it will be the rich and powerful who will avail themselves of them," warns Seamus O'Mahony, a retired Irish physician and the author of *The Way We Die Now*. "Poor people in Africa, Asia, and South America will continue to struggle for simple necessities, such as food, clean water, and basic health care."

We face a moral imperative: ensuring life is every bit as inclusive as it is long for as many as possible in our extended family of nations. After all, "the greatest escape in human history," Nobel economics laureate Angus Deaton once wrote, "is the escape from poverty and death."

I'll confess I'm not sure how we go about closing the longevity gap. Nor am I naïve about the chances of ordinary people of goodwill succeeding where governments, aid workers, and billionaire philanthropists have failed. I just know my 103-year-old grandmother would have done anything—*everything*—in her power to help my uncle, her son, live longer than forty-seven.

As the nineteenth-century writer Christian Nestell Bovee said: "When all else is lost, the future still remains."

Kierkegaard put it even more poignantly: "The most painful state of being is remembering the future"—finding ourselves haunted by all that could have been.

We must build that future together—as individuals, as nations, as rapidly graying fellow inhabitants of an inexorably aging planet.

We all breathe the same air, and we all want the same things: Long, healthy, prosperous, and fulfilling lives free of inequity and injustice. Lives well-lived, in the company of family and friends well-loved. Lives as abundant as they are meaningful, enriching societies that in turn will offer each of us more brightness than bleakness. This book is my attempt at mapping out a path to that future—a *Geezer's Guide to the Galaxy*, if you will.

First things first: We'll never get to where we want to go without understanding where we've been. Over millennia, science, as we've seen, has multiplied our life span several times over. Yet it's being undermined and attacked in our supposedly enlightened modern era by climate change deniers, anti-vaxxers, and extremists of various stripes more interested in banning or burning books than in ingesting knowledge. If we're still not acknowledging the veracity of global warming and our complicity in it, how on earth will we take on the more abstract challenges of a rapidly graying population?

Let's reserve our skepticism for where it's really needed: figuring out the thorny ethics of radical life extension, such as the 3D printing of replacement body parts, and the vexing debate over the growing intelligence and intrusiveness of AI.

Death, it is said, is the great equalizer. Except it's not if it comes so much later to whites and Asians than to Blacks, Latinos, and indigenous people. There are no easy answers here, but we can't give up. In the United States, our spirited nationwide reckoning around race provides an opportunity. It's time to add diminished life expectancy for people of color to the growing list of inequities we're tackling. If we're willing to consider cash reparations to the descendants of slaves, as some cities are doing, we can at least have honest conversations about why some of our friends and neighbors are dying prematurely. We hold these truths to be self-evident: Life is life, and Black and brown people are no less deserving.

Ageism is arguably the most prevalent of all the -isms, crossing racial and ethnic lines, yet there are glimmers of hope shining through the fog of our collective denial. Consider this evocative example in Australia, where high school students are working to close the age gap through an initiative called the Centenarian Portrait Project. Budding artists are paired with 100-year-olds, and they get to know one another as the teens paint or sketch the elders. It's simple, inspired, and beautiful.

Congress desperately needs to repair the federal Age Discrimination in Employment Act that the US Supreme Court inexplicably gutted in 2009. It is unconscionable in a civilized society to insist that people produce more evidence of age bias than what they'd need for a case involving racial, religious, or gender discrimination. Write your representatives and senators, and tell them you expect them to fix this now.

And while you're writing your congressperson, demand they address the liquidity of Social Security. As we've seen, the financial reserves that underpin Social Security are projected to become depleted by 2034 if Congress doesn't act. The approaches we hear about the most—increase payroll taxes, decrease benefits, raise the retirement age, or do some combination of those things—ignore the obvious solution: Make the wealthiest of the wealthy pay their fair share of taxes. Most Americans pay 6.2 percent of their earnings into Social Security. For the rich, the effective tax rate is substantially lower—less than a tenth of a percent in some instances. The Social Security payroll tax cap for 2024 was $168,600, meaning a millionaire hit the limit and stopped paying before the end of February, while most of the rest of us continued to contribute through the end of the year. "The burden of Social Security taxes falls more heavily on those who make less," the Center for Economic Policy Research says.

None of us should be okay with that. It's worse than unfair—it's immoral. Fortunately, some lawmakers are working to right these kinds of wrongs. The US Senate has crafted the Comprehensive Care for Alzheimer's Act, which reenvisions the way Medicare pays for dementia care.

Loneliness theoretically may ease when we eventually hit the stage of our longevity evolution where large numbers of us are reaching 100 together. But we're not there yet, leaving millions of seniors to languish in solitude. Americans could take a cue from the Canadians and replicate Vancouver's innovative "Hey, Neighbor" initiative, where someone in every apartment is paid a stipend to keep close tabs on elderly tenants. We must not forget seniors isolated in private homes or nursing facilities, especially in rural areas. Consider volunteering with your local Council on Aging or "adopting" a childless nursing home resident. Even a twenty-minute visit will brighten their day, and having our eyes and ears inside any given facility will help prevent abuse or neglect.

Merely because seniors are a faithful and formidable voting bloc doesn't mean they're entitled to a lock on government or its resources. As society ages, we need to be mindful of the needs of younger citizens. Just as we'll all be old one day, we'll all have been young: paying for an education, launching a career, buying a home, and raising a family. Our seasons of life are not mutually exclusive. Building an equitable social order means everyone—young *and* old—has access to what they need, including the levers of power. Mandatory mental competency tests for aging politicians are unreasonable. Term limits are not.

"Younger millennials and certainly Gen Z still have some maturation to do before they can properly assume control of national life," Jack Butler, a twenty-something journalist, writes in a commentary for the conservative *National Review*. "Gen X seems well-positioned to steer it next. If, that is, older generations ever get out the door."

Okay, boomer?

The caregiving crisis is acute, but it's also solvable. At a time when birth rates are flat or at best incrementally increasing, as they are in the United States, immigration is the most obvious answer. Never before in human history have so many refugees and migrants been on the move. In my city, there's a sizable population of Central Americans, and I've always been amazed at how readily some—within a few years of their own arrival—clamor for the door to be shut to future newcomers. If we can find a way to overcome our inherent xenophobia and employ immigrants, nearly all of whom are desperate to work, we won't have a caregiver shortage.

Ideally, we'd enact reforms on a federal level and work harder to safely open our borders to sensible levels of immigration. But since bipartisan support for immigration issues is virtually nonexistent, there's nothing stopping "sanctuary states" like California, Oregon, and my native Massachusetts—or "sanctuary cities" like Chicago,

New York, and Washington, DC—from protecting those who are in the country illegally simply to earn a living.

And making a living is something else we all have in common. Changing policy to meet the challenges of our coming 100-year life spans is the government's responsibility. But ensuring we have the foresight to save enough money to last a century or more? That's on us. In a world now largely devoid of pensions and driven by a growing gig economy, it won't be easy. It *is* doable, though. We just have to stop thinking of professional financial advice as something we do in our fifties—and start saving for our nineties and 100s when we're in our twenties or thirties.

Above all, we must renew the optimism that produced China's golden age Tang dynasty, Europe's Renaissance and Enlightenment, and the lively and ever-evolving American experiment. Having an extra decade or two added to a life span has many consequences, some of which likely haven't even occurred to us yet, but one obvious outcome is that we'll have more time to figure it all out.

We got this.

It's okay if we don't have all the answers. What matters most, as we gird for action, is that we're asking the right questions. Today, as our new era of super-aging dawns, let us invoke Pulitzer Prize–winning poet Mary Oliver's "The Summer Day":

> *Doesn't everything die at last, and too soon?*
> *Tell me, what is it you plan to do*
> *With your one wild and precious life?*

THE MOST IMPORTANT THINGS

It's November 15, 2060, and life is . . . what? Good? Not great. But also nowhere near as bad as it could have been.

President Alexandria Ocasio-Cortez cruised to an easy reelection last week. At seventy, some still think she's a little young for the White House—she never did manage to shed that label—but her Green Party and the Climate Coalition made easy work of what's left of the America First-ers.

Not that they'll have much time or reason to celebrate. Although Earth is still largely livable, parts of the planet are every bit the shitshow we were warned about.

World leaders were supposed to gather on Cape Cod next month for the biennial UN climate change summit, but COP46 had to be hastily relocated to Reykjavik after half of the peninsula sank from view. Now, with the rising North Atlantic pushing ever inland, United Nations Secretary-General Greta Thunberg says the talks may have to be moved again.

Half a century ago, many of us thought by now we'd be colonizing Mars, but sadly, 2060 is far more like *Waterworld* than *Interstellar*.

At least our last seven presidents, like the other leaders of the G7, have all been women. As Pope Maria IV says, their steely resolve in rising above nationalism and petty politics to embrace and defend Mother Earth has kept us—for now, anyway—off the endangered species list.

As for me? I turned the big 100 today.

Sure, I've slowed down. My marathon times are a joke. But I'm grateful for these years; for my health; and above all for my family. It took me more of my century than I'd care to admit to fully appreciate the most important things: love and laughter.

When I was born in 1960, total life expectancy for an American was 69.7 years. A hundred years later, it's at an all-time high of 85.6 years—exactly what the US Census Bureau had projected way back in the 2020s. But that's just a number. Now that I've finally joined the rising ranks of centenarians, I'll let you in on a little secret: So is 100.

Exceptionally long, tragically short, or something in between, life is sweet, and we only get one shot at getting it right. As our new US poet laureate, Taylor Swift, sang so long ago:

> I have this thing where I get older but just never wiser . . .
> It's me, hi, I'm the problem, it's me.

ACKNOWLEDGMENTS

It takes a village to raise a child. The same could certainly be said of writing a book.

I'll be forever grateful to my wife, Terry DeYonker Kole, and my children, Nicholas and Erin, for their enthusiastic support. It was you, E., whose early mention of the horrifically unjust phenomenon of "weathering" prompted me to take a closer look at how systemic racism affects aging in communities of color.

Special thanks to agents Rick Richter and Caroline Marsiglia at Aevitas Creative Management for taking a chance on me as a new author. You believed in me and this project, and tirelessly helped me refine the concept in ways big and small.

I've never met a writer who wasn't in desperate need of an editor, and I'm so very thankful for Keith Wallman at Diversion Books, whose deft hand and creative vision vastly improved these pages. Deepest thanks, too, to Evan Phail, Clara Linhoff, Jane Glaser, Shannon Donnelly, and Alex Sprague at Diversion for patiently helping this newbie navigate the many twists and turns of the publishing process, and to designer Jonathan Sainsbury for his magic with the cover.

Two treasured colleagues at the Associated Press—Mallika Sen and Alanna Durkin Richer—provided invaluable feedback in the early going as I sought to hit the right notes and settle on the proper frame for the ground that's covered in this book. Thank you both.

Grazie mille to one of my dearest and oldest (sorry) pals, Brian Murphy of the *Washington Post*—a man whose books I so admire—for the example, the encouragement, and, before I quit drinking, the wine. And a special shout-out to new friend Carlos Enriquez, who spoke into my life precisely at a moment when it looked like this book wouldn't happen and insisted I not take no for an answer. You were right, amigo.

Thanks to the many incredible minds who consented to be interviewed: the indefatigable Dr. Jane Goodall; the irrepressibly witty, 112-year-old supercentenarian Herlda Senhouse; cardiologist and occasional sailing companion Dr. Richard Regnante; Jongseong Lee, an architect of South Korea's impressive national elder care system; and an impressive lineup of other thinkers, activists, caregivers, and policymakers, including Vida Bampoe; Anne Basting; John Beard; Mary Ann Evan; Bill McKibben; Wendy McRae-Owoeye; Martin Picard; and Beth Truesdale.

Heartfelt appreciation to the National Press Foundation, especially Sonni Efron and Rachel Jones, and to Caitlin Hawke of Columbia University. Your brilliantly organized fellowships for journalists covering aging issues put me face-to-face, in Washington and online, with a litany of experts whose perspectives enliven this book: Jean Accius, William Beach, Martha Boudreau, Catherine Collinson, Joseph Coughlin, Robert Espinoza, Ruth Finkelstein, Cristina Martin Firvida, Linda Fried, Joseph Fuller, Peter Gosselin, David Grabowski, Patti Greco, Paul Irving, David John, Greg Link, Ai-jen Poo, Siavash Radpour, Susan Reinhard, Jason Resendez, Sheria Robinson-Lane, John Schall, Derenda Schubert, Brian Smedley, Robyn Stone, Yulya Truskinovsky, Debra Whitman, and Jennifer Wolff.

Cheers to erstwhile commuting buddy David Schultz, who told me about his 106-year-old great-grandfather, and to a trio of journalists I admire who contributed in passing but profound ways they probably aren't even aware of: Norm Abelson, Mort Rosenblum, and Peter Prengaman. To others whose names I've omitted, please accept my appreciation and my apologies. You can blame my advancing age.

My deepest gratitude must be reserved for Dr. Thomas T. Perls, founder and director of the New England Centenarian Study. We bonded over our shared fascination with Jeanne Calment and other supercentenarians, and it's no exaggeration to say your brain powers the entire arc of this narrative. There'd be no book without you, Tom.

Last, to my centenarian grandmother, Marie Mercurio Sansone, and my sweet nonagenarian mother, Marie "Nadine" Kole, thank you for literally everything: life itself. *Alla famiglia, signore!*

BIBLIOGRAPHY

BOOKS

Berkman, Lisa F., and Beth C. Truesdale. *Overtime: America's Aging Workforce and the Future of Working Longer.* London: Oxford University Press, 2022.

Bradford, William. *Of Plimouth Plantation.* Boston: 1630.

Buckley, Christopher. *Boomsday.* New York: Twelve, Hachette Book Group, 2007.

Coughlin, Joseph. *The Longevity Economy: Unlocking the World's Fastest-Growing, Most Misunderstood Market.* New York: Public Affairs, 2017.

Oliver, Mary. *House of Light.* Boston: Beacon Press, 1990.

Shatner, William, with Joshua Brandon. *Boldly Go.* New York: Simon & Schuster, 2022.

Tolstoy, Leo. *Anna Karenina.* Moscow: T. Ris, 1878.

Van Dyke, Dick. *Keep Moving.* New York: Hachette Books, 2015.

JOURNAL ARTICLES

Almeida, D. M., J. Rush, J. Mogle, J.R. Piazza, E. Cerino, S.T. Charles. "Longitudinal Change in Daily Stress Across 20 Years of Adulthood: Results From the National Study of Daily Experiences." *Developmental Psychology* (November 30, 2022). https://doi.org/10.1037/dev0001469.

Andersen, Stacy L. "Centenarians as Models of Resistance and Resilience to Alzheimer's Disease and Related Dementias." *Advances in Geriatric Medicine and Research* (July 30, 2020). https://doi.org/10.20900/agmr20200018.

Araújo, Lia, Laetitia Teixeira, Rosa Marina Afonso, Oscar Ribeiro. "To Live or Die: What to Wish at 100 Years and Older." *Frontiers in Psychology* (September 10, 2021). https://doi.org/10.3389/fpsyg.2021.726621.

Atella, Vincenzo, and Lorenzo Carbonari, "Is Gerontocracy Harmful for Growth? A Comparative Study of Seven European Countries." *Journal of Applied Economics* (January 22, 2019). http://dx.doi.org/10.1016/S1514 -0326(17)30007-7.

Banerjee, Abhijit V., and Esther Duflo. "The Economic Lives of the Poor." *Journal of Economic Perspectives* (October 2006). https://doi.org/10.1257/jep.21.1.141.

Beker, Nina, Andrea Ganz, Marc Hulsman, Henne Holstege. "Association of Cognitive Function Trajectories in Centenarians with Postmortem Neuropathology, Physical Health, and Other Risk Factors for Cognitive Decline." *Journal of the American Medical Association* (January 15, 2021). https://doi.org/10.1001%2Fjamanetworkopen.2020.31654.

Brandts, Lloyd, Theo G. van Tilburg, Hans Bosma, Martijn Huisman, Piet A. van den Brandt. "Loneliness in Later Life and Reaching Longevity: Findings from the Longitudinal Aging Study Amsterdam." *Journals of Gerontology* (February 2021). https://doi.org/10.1093/geronb/gbaa145.

Cagan, Alex, Adrian Baez-Ortega, Natalia Brzozowska, Federico Abascal, Tim H. H. Coorens, Mathijs A. Sanders, Andrew R. J. Lawson, Luke M. R. Harvey, Shriram Bhosle, David Jones. "Somatic Mutation Rates Scale with Lifespan across Mammals." *Nature* (April 13, 2022). https://doi.org/10.1038/s41586-022-04618-z.

Case, Anne, and Angus Deaton. "Life Expectancy in Adulthood Is Falling for Those without a BA Degree." *Proceedings of the National Academy of Sciences* (March 8, 2021). https://doi.org/10.1073%2Fpnas.2024777118.

Chapman, Susan A., Lillie Greiman, Timothy Bates, Laura M. Wagner, Ari Lissau, Kirsi Toivanen-Atilla, Rayna Sage. "Assessing Self-Care Needs and Worker Shortages in Rural Areas." *Health Affairs* (October 2022). https://doi.org/10.1377/hlthaff.2022.00483.

Costumero, Victor, Lidon Marin-Marin, Marco Calabria, Vicente Belloch, Joaquín Escudero, Miguel Baquero, Mireia Hernandez, Juan Ruiz de Miras, Albert Costa, Maria-Antònia Parcet & César Ávila. "A Cross-Sectional and Longitudinal Study on the Protective Effect of Bilingualism against Dementia." *Alzheimer's Research & Therapy* (January 10, 2020). https://doi.org/10.1186%2Fs13195-020-0581-1.

Cox, John. "Joe Smith: Centenarian Refuses to Leave His Job after 57 Years at Same Firm." *Bakersfield Californian*, August 2, 2022. https://www.bakersfield.com/news/centenarian-refuses-to-leave-his-job-after-57-years-at-same-firm/article_08cf1caa-12ba-11ed-8248-7bfbb2eb6e1c.html.

Crane, Keith, Roger Cliff, Evan S. Medeiros, James C. Mulvenon, William H. Overholt. "Forecasting China's Military Spending Through 2025." *RAND Corp.*, 2005. https://doi.org/10.7249/RB162.

Daniel, Caitlin. "Is Healthy Food Too Expensive?" *American Sociological Association* (March 2021). https://www.asanet.org/wp-content/uploads/attach/footnotes/footnotes-winter_2021.pdf.

Den Dunnen, Wilfred F.A., Wiebo H. Brouwer, Eveline Bijlard, Jeanine Kamphuis, Klaas van Linschoten, Ellie Eggens-Meijer, Gert Holstege. "No Disease in the Brain of a 115-Year-Old Woman." *Neurobiology of Aging* (August 2008). https://doi.org/10.1016/j.neurobiolaging.2008.04.010.

Ding, Ding, Joe Van Buskirk, Binh Nguyen, Emmanuel Stamatakis, Mona Elbarbary, Nicola Veronese, Philip J. Clare, Min Lee, Ulf Ekelund, Luigi

Fontana. "Physical Activity, Diet Quality and All-Cause Cardiovascular Disease and Cancer Mortality." *British Journal of Sports Medicine* (July 8, 2022). https://doi.org/10.1136/bjsports-2021-105195.

Dong, XinQi. "Elder Rights in China: Care for Your Parents or Suffer Public Shaming." *JAMA* (October 1, 2016). https://doi.org/10.1001/jamainternmed .2016.5011.

Drew, Liam. "Turning Back Time with Epigenetic Clocks." *Nature* (January 19, 2022). https://www.nature.com/articles/d41586-022-00077-8.

Farrell, Timothy W., William W. Hung, Kathleen T. Unroe, Teneille R. Brown, Christian D. Furman, Jane Jih, Reena Karani, Paul Mulhausen, Anna María Nápoles, Joseph O. Nnodim, et al. "Exploring the Intersection of Structural Racism and Ageism in Healthcare." *Journal of the American Geriatrics Society* (October 19, 2022). https://doi.org/10.1111/jgs.18105.

Fishman, Ezra. "Risk of Developing Dementia at Older Ages in the United States." *Demography* (August 3, 2017). https://doi.org/10.1007%2Fs13524 -017-0598-7.

Fukuda, Takafumia, Tohrub Ohnuma, Kuniakia Obara, Sumioc Kondo, Heeib Arai, Yasuhisa Ano. "Supplementation with Matured Hop Bitter Acids Improves Cognitive Performance and Mood State in Healthy Older Adults with Subjective Cognitive Decline." *Journal of Alzheimer's Disease* (June 30, 2020). https://doi.org/10.3233/JAD-200229.

Geronimus, Arline T. "Dying Old at a Young Age from Pre-Existing Racist Conditions." *Washington and Lee Journal of Civil Rights and Social Justice* (Spring 2021). https://scholarlycommons.law.wlu.edu/crsj/vol27/iss2/5.

Geronimus, Arline T., Margaret T. Hicken, Jay A. Pearson, Sarah J. Seashols, Kelly L. Brown & Tracey Dawson Cruz. "Do US Black Women Experience Stress-Related Accelerated Biological Aging?" *Human Nature* (March 11, 2010). https://doi.org/10.1007%2Fs12110-010-9078-0.

Gutin, Iliya, Robert A. Hummer. "Social Inequality and the Future of US Life Expectancy." *Annual Review of Sociology* (March 10, 2021). https://doi .org/10.1146/annurev-soc-072320-100249.

Holland, Thomas Monroe, Puja Agarwal, Yamin Wang, Klodian Dhana, Sue E. Leurgans, Kyla Shea, Sarah L Booth, Kumar Rajan, Julie A. Schneider, Lisa L. Barnes, et al. "Association of Dietary Intake of Flavonols with Changes in Global Cognition and Several Cognitive Abilities." *Neurology* (November 22, 2022). https://doi.org/10.1212/WNL.0000000000201541.

Holt-Lunstad, Julianne, Timothy B. Smith, David Stephenson. "Loneliness and Social Isolation as Risk Factors for Mortality." *Perspectives on Psychological Science* (March 11, 2015). https://doi.org/10.1177/1745691614568352.

Inglés, Marta, Angel Belenguer-Varea, Eva Serna, Cristina Mas-Bargues, Francisco J. Tarazona-Santabalbina, Consuelo Borrás, Jose Vina. "Analysis of Centenarians' Offspring Reveals a Specific Genetic Footprint." *Journals of Gerontology* (May 28, 2022). https://doi.org/10.1093/gerona/glac119.

Jia, Haomiao, Erica I. Lubetkin. "Life Expectancy and Active Life Expectancy by Marital Status among Older U.S. Adults: Results From the U.S. Medicare Health Outcome Survey." *SSM Population Health* (December 12, 2020). https://doi.org/10.1016%2Fj.ssmph.2020.100642

Jopp, Daniela. "Aging Researcher: 'At 100, Health Problems Are No Longer So Important.'" *Profil* (December 12, 2022). https://www.profil.at/wissenschaft/alternsforscherin-daniela-jopp-im-interview/402253695.

Jopp, Daniela, Charikleia Lampraki, Dario Spini. "Heterogeneity in Vulnerability and Resilience Among Centenarians." *Innovation in Aging* (December 17, 2021). https://doi.org/10.1093%2Fgeroni%2Figab046.415.

Katsimpardi, Lida, Nadia K. Litterman, Panela A. Schein, Christine M. Miller, Francesco S. Loffredo, Gregory R. Wojtkiewicz, John W. Chen, Richard T. Lee, Amy J. Wagers, Lee L. Rubin. "Vascular and Neurogenic Rejuvenation of the Aging Mouse Brain by Young Systemic Factors." *Science* (May 9, 2014). https://doi.org/10.1126/science.1251141.

Kim, Yevgeniy, Zharylkasyn Zharkinbekov, Madina Sarsenova, Gaziza Yeltay, Arman Saparov . "Advances in Gene Therapy." *International Journal of Molecular Sciences* (August 26, 2021). https://doi.org/10.3390/ijms22179206.

Koga, Hayami K., Claudia Trudel-Fitzgerald, Lewina O. Lee, Peter James, Candyce Kroenke, Lorena Garcia, Aladdin H. Shadyab, Elena Salmoirago-Blotcher, JoAnn E. Manson, Francine Grodstein et al. "Optimism, Lifestyle, and Longevity in a Racially Diverse Cohort of Women." *Journal of the American Geriatrics Society* (April 23, 2022). https://doi.org/10.1111/jgs.17897.

Kreouzi, Magdalini, Nikolaos Theodorakis, Constantina Constantinou. "Lessons Learned from Blue Zones, Lifestyle Medicine Pillars and Beyond: An Update on the Contributions of Behavior and Genetics to Wellbeing and Longevity." *American Journal of Lifestyle Medicine* (August 20, 2022). https://doi.org/10.1177/15598276221118494.

Lee, Lewina O., Francine Grodstein, Claudia Trudel-Fitzgerald, Peter James, Sakurako S. Okuzono, Hayami K. Koga, Joel Schwartz, Avron Spiro III, Daniel K Mroczek, Laura D. Kubzansky. "Optimism, Daily Stressors, and Emotional Well-Being Over Two Decades in a Cohort of Aging Men." *Journals of Gerontology* (March 7, 2022). https://doi.org/10.1093/geronb/gbaco25.

Leitch, Sharon, Paul Glue, Andrew R. Gray. "Comparison of Psychosocial Variables Associated with Loneliness in Centenarian vs Elderly Populations in New Zealand." *JAMA Network* (October 26, 2018). https://doi.org/10.1001/jamanetworkopen.2018.3880.

Levy, Becca R., Martin D. Slade, Stanislav V. Kasl. "Longitudinal Benefit of Positive Self-Perceptions of Aging on Functional Health." *Journals of Gerontology* (September 1, 2002). https://doi.org/10.1093/geronb/57.5.p409.

Li, Shanshan, Meir J. Stampfer, David R. Williams. "Association of Religious Service Attendance with Mortality Among Women." *JAMA Internal Medicine* (June 2016). https://doi.org/10.1001/jamainternmed.2016.1615.

Lipka, Michael. "A Closer Look at Seventh-day Adventists in America." Pew Research Center (November 3, 2015). https://www.pewresearch.org/fact-tank /2015/11/03/a-closer-look-at-seventh-day-adventists-in-america/.

Lu, Yuancheng, Benedikt Brommer, Xiao Tian, Anitha Krishnan, Margarita Meer, Chen Wang, Daniel L. Vera, Qiurui Zeng, Doudou Yu, Michael S. Bonkowski, et al. "Reprogramming to Recover Youthful Epigenetic Information and Restore Vision." *Nature* (December 2, 2020). https://doi .org/10.1038/s41586-020-2975-4.

Melenhorst, J. Joseph, Gregory M. Chen, Meng Wang, David L. Porter, Changya Chen, McKensie A. Collins, Peng Gao, Shovik Bandyopadhyay, Hongxing Sun, et al. "Decade-Long Leukaemia Remissions with Persistence of CD4+ CAR T Cells." *Nature* (February 2, 2022). https://doi.org/10.1038/s41586-021-04390-6.

Milholland, Brandon, Jan Vijg. "Why Gilgamesh Failed: The Mechanistic Basis of the Limits to Human Lifespan." *Nature Aging* (October 14, 2022). https://doi .org/10.1038/s43587-022-00291-z.

Newman, Saul Justin. "Supercentenarians and the Oldest-Old Are Concentrated Into Regions with No Birth Certificates and Short Lifespans." *bioRxiv* (July 16, 2019). https://doi.org/10.1101/704080.

Olshansky, S. Jay. "From Lifespan to Healthspan." *JAMA* (October 2, 2018). https://doi.org/10.1001/jama.2018.12621.

Olshansky S. Jay, Bruce A. Carnes. "Inconvenient Truths About Human Longevity." *Journals of Gerontology* (April 19, 2019). https://doi.org/10.1093 /gerona/glz098.

Palmioli, Alessandro, Valeria Mazzoni, Ada De Luigi, Chiara Bruzzone, Gessica Sala, Laura Colombo, Chiara Bazzini, Chiara Paola Zoia, Mariagiovanna Inserra, Mario Salmona, et al. "Alzheimer's Disease Prevention Through Natural Compounds." *American Chemical Society/Neuroscience* (October 25, 2022). https://doi.org/10.1021/acschemneuro.2c00444.

Pearce, Michael, Adrian E. Raftery. "Probabilistic Forecasting of Maximum Human Lifespan by 2100 Using Bayesian Population Projections." *Demographic Research* (June 30, 2021). https://doi.org/10.4054/DemRes.2021.44.52.

Pijnenburg, Martien, Carlo Leget. "Who Wants to Live Forever? Three Arguments against Extending the Human Lifespan." *Journal of Medical Ethics* (October 2007). https://doi.org/10.1136%2Fjme.2006.017822.

Pillai, Jagan A., Charles B. Hall, Dennis W. Dickson, Herman Buschke, Richard B. Lipton, Joe Verghese. "Association of Crossword Puzzle Participation with Memory Decline in Persons Who Develop Dementia." *Journal of the International Neuropsychological Society* (September 28, 2011). https://doi .org/10.1017/S1355617711001111.

Podolskiy, Dmitriy I., Andrei Avanesov, Alexander Tyshkovskiy, Emily Porter, Michael Petrascheck, Matt Kaeberlein, Vadim N. Gladyshev. "The Landscape of Longevity across Phylogeny." *bioRxiv* (March 17, 2020). https://doi .org/10.1101/2020.03.17.995993.

Preston, Samuel H., Irma T. Elo. "Black Mortality at Very Old Ages." *Population and Development Review* (September 8, 2006). http://dx.doi .org/10.1111/j.1728-4457.2006.00137.x.

Pyrkov, Timothy V., Konstantin Avchaciov, Andrei E. Tarkhov, Leonid I. Menshikov, Andrei V. Gudkov, Peter O. Fedichev. "Longitudinal Analysis of Blood Markers Reveals Progressive Loss of Resilience and Predicts Human Lifespan Limit." *Nature Communications* (May 25, 2021). https://doi .org/10.1038/s41467-021-23014-1.

Quiroz, Yakeel T., Michele Solis, María P. Aranda, Alicia I. Arbaje, Mirna Arroyo-Miranda, Laura Y. Cabrera, Minerva Maria Carrasquillo, Maria M. Corrada, Lucia Crivelli, Erica D. Diminich. "Alzheimer's in Latinx Population: Addressing the Disparities in Dementia Risk, Early Detection and Care in Latino Populations." *Alzheimer's & Dementia* (September 18, 2022). https://doi.org/10.1002/alz.12589.

Ribeiro, Oscar, Laetitia Teixeira, Lia Araújo, Rosa Marina Afonso, Nancy Pachana. "Predictors of Anxiety in Centenarians: Health, Economic Factors, and Loneliness." Cambridge University Press (August 13, 2014). https://www.cambridge.org/core/journals/international-psychogeriatrics /article/abs/predictors-of-anxiety-in-centenarians-health-economic -factors-and-loneliness/C24DD58D2410A894C15910DADA7B6A55.

Robine, Jean-Marie, Michel Allard, Francois R. Herrmann, Bernard Jeune. "The Real Facts Supporting Jeanne Calment as the Oldest Ever Human." *Journals of Gerontology* (September 16, 2019). https://doi.org/10.1093/gerona/glz198.

Rogalski, Emily. "What Makes Someone a SuperAger?" *Feinberg School of Medicine podcast* (August 28, 2018). https://www.feinberg.northwestern.edu/research /news/podcast/what-makes-someone-a-superager.html.

Schafer, Markus H., Haosen Sun, Jin A. Lee. "Compensatory Connections? Living Alone, Loneliness, and the Buffering Role of Social Connection Among Older American and European Adults." *Journals of Gerontology* (August 8, 2022). https://doi.org/10.1093/geronb/gbab217.

Schwandt, Hannes, Janet Currie, Marlies Bär, Amelie Wuppermann. "Life Expectancy Gap between Races: Inequality in Mortality between Black and White Americans by Age, Place, and Cause and in Comparison to Europe, 1990 to 2018." *Proceedings of the National Academy of Sciences* (September 28, 2021). https://doi.org/10.1073/pnas.2104684118.

Staff, Roger T., Michael J. Hogan, Daniel S. Williams, L. J. Whalley. "Intellectual Engagement and Cognitive Ability in Later Life." *British Medical Journal* (December 10, 2018). https://doi.org/10.1136/bmj.k4925.

Su, Sizhen, Le Shi, Yongbo Zheng, Yankun Sun, Xiaolin Huang, Anyi Zhang, Jianyu Que, Xinyu Sun, Jie Shi, Yanping Bao, Jiahui Deng, Lin Lu. "Leisure Activities and the Risk of Dementia: A Systematic Review and Meta-Analysis." *Neurology* (August 10, 2022). https://doi.org/10.1212/WNL .0000000000200929.

Vacante, Marco, Velia D'Agata, Massimo Motta, Giulia Malaguarnera, Antonio Biondi, Francesco Basile, Michele Malaguarnera, Caterina Gagliano, Filippo Drago, Salvatore Salamone. "Centenarians and Supercentenarians: A Black Swan." *BMC Surgery* (November 15, 2012). https://doi.org/10.1186/1471-2482 -12-S1-S36.

Wallace, Laura E., Rebecca Anthony, Baldwin M. Way. "Does Religion Stave Off the Grave? Religious Affiliation in One's Obituary and Longevity." *Social Psychological and Personality Science* (June 13, 2018). https://doi .org/10.1177/1948550618779820.

Wang, Lindsey, Pamela Davis, Nora Volkow, Nathan Berger, David Kaelber, Rong Xu. "Association of COVID-19 with New-Onset Alzheimer's Disease." *Journal of Alzheimer's Disease* (September 16, 2022). https://doi.org/10.3233 /jad-220717.

Wong, Serena, Kenneth I. Pargament, Carol Ann Faigin. "Sustained by the Sacred: Religious and Spiritual Factors for Resilience in Adulthood and Aging: Concepts, Research, and Outcomes." *Resilience in Aging*, January 2018: http://dx.doi.org/10.1007/978-3-030-04555-5_10.

Wu, Lei, Xinqiang Xie, Ying Li, Tingting Liang, Haojie Zhong, Lingshuang Yang, Yu Xi, Jumei Zhang, Yu Ding, Qingping Wu. "Gut Microbiota as an Antioxidant System in Centenarians." *Nature* (December 24, 2022). https://doi.org/10.1038 /s41522-022-00366-0.

Xu, Chi, Timothy A. Kohler, Timothy M. Lenton, Marten Scheffer. "Future of the Human Climate Niche." *Proceedings of the National Academy of Sciences of the United States of America* (May 4, 2020). https://doi.org/10.1073/pnas.1910114117.

Young, Robert Douglas. "African American Longevity Advantage: Myth or Reality? A Racial Comparison of Supercentenarian Data." *Georgia State University ScholarWorks* (July 21, 2008). https://scholarworks.gsu.edu/cgi /viewcontent.cgi?article=1009&context=gerontology_theses.

Zhu, Jianwei, Fenfen Ge, Yu Zeng, Yuanyuan Qu, Wenwen Chen, Huazhen Yang, Lei Yang, Fang Fang, Huan Song. "Physical and Mental Activity, Disease Susceptibility, and Risk of Dementia: A Prospective Cohort Study Based on UK Biobank." *Neurology* (July 27, 2022). https://doi.org/10.1212/WNL .0000000000200701.

NEWSPAPER AND MAGAZINE ARTICLES

"A 120-Year Lease on Life Outlasts Apartment Heir." *New York Times*, December 29, 1995.

"Angela Lansbury Adds Another Role: ALS Spokeswoman." Associated Press, April 15, 2008.

"Dagny Carlsson, Centenarian Blogger, Dies at Age 109." Associated Press, March 25, 2022: https://apnews.com/article/europe-lifestyle-media-stockholm-sweden-f8630ad1fe716e49075629cb6da51d33.

"Friends, Admirers Pay Tribute to Life of World's Oldest Person." Associated Press, August 7, 1997.

"Jeanne Calment, World's Oldest Person, Dead at 122." Associated Press, August 4, 1997.

"Living Next to Water Could Make You Live Longer: Study." CBC News, July 27, 2018. https://www.cbc.ca/news/canada/new-brunswick/living-water-reduced-risk-dying-unb-study-1.4763647.

"Mimi Reinhard, Who Typed up Schindler's List, Dies at 107." Associated Press, April 11, 2022. https://apnews.com/article/business-israel-middle-east-steven-spielberg-poland-c1efdb74160288ae7caacffdfa806b38.

"1 of Nation's Oldest Farmers Gives Lesson on Longevity." ABC News, August 21, 2022. https://abcnews.go.com/WNT/video/nations-oldest-farmers-lesson-longevity-88670271.

"Virginia McLaurin, Who Danced with the Obamas, Dies at 113." Associated Press, November 15, 2022. https://apnews.com/article/michelle-obama-barack-obituaries-33c82cda5c239f1e4c99a1ba0229341d.

"What Is a Brain-Healthy Lifestyle? How to Protect, Improve Cognition." *TODAY Show*, November 3, 2022. https://www.youtube.com/watch?v=eYFJS25cMos.

"Wesley Brown, Nation's Oldest Federal Judge, Dies at Age 104." Associated Press, January 24, 2012. https://www.politico.com/story/2012/01/wesley-brown-nations-oldest-federal-judge-dies-at-age-104-071888.

Abelson, Norm. "Ageism Infects Politics." *Connecting*, Nov. 23, 2022.

Anderson, Curt. "Exuberant Springsteen, E St. Band Launch 1st Tour in 6 Years." Associated Press, February 2, 2023. https://apnews.com/article/celebrity-music-entertainment-tampa-19eb75b89815edb52b78a8dfdf27c1e4.

Alvarez, Alayna. "Jane Goodall Exhibit Headed to Denver Museum of Nature & Science." *Axios*, March 29, 2023. https://www.axios.com/local/denver/2023/03/29/jane-goodall-exhibit-denver-museum-of-nature-science.

Bacon, John. "'All I Want Is to Die.' Longest Living Human Ever? Maybe, but Indonesian man dead at 146." *USA Today*, May 2, 2017. https://www.usatoday.com/story/news/world/2017/05/02/longest-living-human-ever-maybe-but-hes-dead-146/101190074/.

Banerjee, Abhijit V., and Esther Duflo. "How Poverty Ends." *Foreign Affairs*, February 2020. https://www.foreignaffairs.com/world/how-poverty-ends.

Birnstengl, Grace. "How'd We Get Here? The History of Nursing Homes." *Next Avenue*, March 5, 2021. https://www.nextavenue.org/history-of-nursing-homes/.

Boak, Josh, and Hannah Fingerhut. "Biden 2024? Most Democrats Say No Thank You: AP-NORC Poll." *AP*, February 6, 2023. https://apnews.com/article/ap-norc -poll-biden-2024-presidential-prospects-c843c5af6775b4c8a0 cff8e2b1db03f6.

Breznican, Anthony. "Chris Hemsworth Changed His Life after an Ominous Health Warning." *Vanity Fair*, November 17, 2022. https://www.vanityfair .com/hollywood/2022/11/chris-hemsworth-exclusive-interview -alzheimers-limitless.

Bryner, Jeanna. "Thanking 'Cigars and God,' Oldest US Vet Turns 111." *Live Science*, May 12, 2017. https://www.livescience.com/59089-oldest-us-veteran -turns-111.html.

Butler, Jack. "The Problem of Gerontocracy." *National Review*, July 1, 2022. https://www.nationalreview.com/corner/the-problem-of-gerontocracy/.

Campbell, Heather, and Eddy Elmer. "Solutions for Chronic Loneliness Need Innovation and Vision." *The Province*, September 8, 2018. https://theprovince .com/opinion/op-ed/heather-campbell-and-eddy-elmer-solutions-for -chronic-loneliness-need-innovation-and-vision.

Carey, Jacqueline. "New Study Finds Biden, Trump Both Likely to Be 'Super-Agers.'" *University of Illinois-Chicago School of Public Health*, September 25, 2020. https://publichealth.uic.edu/news-stories/new-study-finds-biden -trump-both-likely-to-be-super-agers/.

Chappell, Bill. "3 Experts Have Resigned from an FDA Committee over Alzheimer's Drug Approval." *NPR*, June 11, 2021. https://www.npr.org/2021 /06/11/1005567149/3-experts-have-resigned-from-an-fda-committee-over -alzheimers-drug-approval.

Chu, Louise. "Ephraim Engleman, One of World's Oldest Practicing Physicians, Dies at 104." University of California San Francisco, Sept. 4, 2015. https:// www.ucsf.edu/news/2015/09/131496/ephraim-engleman-one-worlds -oldest-practicing-physicians-dies-104.

Daley, Lauren. "Fashion Icon Iris Apfel's Surprising Connection to Salem." WBUR, February 22, 2022. https://www.wbur.org/news/2022/02/22 /iris-apfel-peabody-essex-museum.

Davis, John. K. "Want to Live Longer? Consider the Ethics." *The Conversation*, August 31, 2018. https://theconversation.com/want-to-live-longer -consider-the-ethics-101301.

Della Volpe, John. "Republicans, Fear the Young." *New York Times*, November 19, 2022. https://www.nytimes.com/2022/11/19/opinion/youth -vote-midterm-election.html.

Doolittle, Robyn. "Lisa LaFlamme 'Going Grey' Questioned by CTV Executive, Says Senior Company Official." *The Globe and Mail*, August 18, 2022. https:// www.theglobeandmail.com/canada/article-lisa-laflamme-ctv-grey-hair/.

Ellison, Tom. "I've Optimized My Health to Make My Life as Long and Unpleasant as Possible." *McSweeney's Internet Tendency*, March 3, 2023. https://www

.mcsweeneys.net/articles/ive-optimized-my-health-to-make-my-life-as
-long-and-unpleasant-as-possible

Elmer, Eddy. "Vision 20/20: Social Isolation and Loneliness." *Zoomer Magazine*, March/April 2020. https://www.vancouverseniorsadvisory.ca/wp-content /uploads/Zoomer_Magazine_Eddy_Elmer_March_2020.pdf.

Emanuel, Ezekiel. "Why I Hope to Die at 75." *The Atlantic*, October 2014. https://www.theatlantic.com/magazine/archive/2014/10/why-i-hope-to -die-at-75/379329/.

Epstein, Reid J., and Jennifer Medina. "Should Biden Run in 2024? Democratic Whispers of 'No' Start to Rise." *New York Times*, June 11, 2022. https://www .nytimes.com/2022/06/11/us/politics/biden-2024-election-democrats.html.

Farrell, Chris. "Who'll Pay for Americans to Live to 100?" *Forbes*, February 8, 2016. https://www.forbes.com/sites/nextavenue/2016/02/08/wholl-pay -for-americans-to-live-to-100/?sh=aff964954e67.

Foster, Malcolm. "Aging Japan: Robots May Have Role in Future of Elder Care." Reuters, March 27, 2018. https://www.reuters.com/article /us-japan-ageing-robots-widerimage/aging-japan-robots-may-have-role -in-future-of-elder-care-idUSKBN1H33AB.

Fraser, Jayme, Nick Penzenstadler, Jeff Kelly Lowenstein. "Many Nursing Homes Are Poorly Staffed. How Do They Get Away with It?" *USA Today*, December 2, 2022. https://www.usatoday.com/in-depth/news/investigations/2022/12/01 /skilled-nursing-facilities-staffing-problems-biden-reforms/8318780001/.

Fukada, Shiho. "Japan Faces Its Old Age with Robots and Virtual Reality." *STAT News*, Feb. 5, 2018. https://www.statnews.com/2018/02/05 /aging-japan-robots-virtual-reality/.

Gilbert, Caitlin. "How Does the Brain Age across the Lifespan? New Studies Offer Clues." *Washington Post*, Feb. 28, 2023. https://www.washingtonpost .com/wellness/2023/02/28/brain-aging-childhood-teens-adults/.

Graham, Mackenzie. "Would a Longer Lifespan Make Us Happier? A Philosopher's Take." *The Conversation*, July 18, 2018. https://theconversation .com/would-a-longer-lifespan-make-us-happier-a-philosophers -take-99619.

Greco, Patti. "This Is Our Long Goodbye." *Oh, Balloon*, November 23, 2022. https:// pattigreco.substack.com/p/this-is-our-long-goodbye?utm_source=profile &utm_medium=reader2.

Greshko, Michael. "Historic Moment: Why the WHO Endorsed the First Malaria Vaccine." *National Geographic*, October 7, 2021. https://www .nationalgeographic.com/science/article/why-the-who-endorsed-the-first -malaria-vaccine-and-what-to-expect-next.

Hamzelou, Jessica. "Next up for CRISPR: Gene Editing for the Masses?" *MIT Technology Review*, January 19, 2023. https://www.technologyreview .com/2023/01/19/1067074/next-for-crispr/.

Harrar, Sari. "It's Time to Throw Out Stereotypes on Aging." *AARP*, June 6, 2022. https://www.aarp.org/health/healthy-living/info-2022/aging-survey.html.

Hathaway, Bill. "Stress Makes Life's Clock Tick Faster—Chilling Out Slows It Down." *Yale News*, December 6, 2021. https://news.yale.edu/2021/12/06 /stress-makes-lifes-clock-tick-faster-chilling-out-slows-it-down.

Hida, Hikari, John Yoon. "In a Japanese Nursing Home, Some Workers Are Babies." *New York Times*, September 1, 2022. https://www.nytimes .com/2022/09/01/world/asia/japan-nursing-home-babies.html.

Higgs, Paul, Chris Gilleard. "Who Wants to Live to a Hundred?" *The Conversation*, June 28, 2018. https://theconversation.com/who-wants-to-live-to -a-hundred-98357.

Hilliard, John. "After a Lifetime of Learning, a 92-Year-Old Newton Woman Earns Her College Degree." *Boston Globe* (May 18, 2022). https://www.bostonglobe .com/2022/05/18/metro/after-lifetime-learning-92-year-old-newton -woman-earns-her-college-degree/.

Horowitz, Jason. "Francis, Slowed by Aging, Finds Lessons in Frailty." *New York Times*, July 28, 2022. https://www.nytimes.com/2022/07/28/world/americas /pope-francis-canada-elderly.html.

Inada, Miho. "In Aging Japan, Under 75 Is the New 'Pre-Old.'" *Wall Street Journal*, September 24, 2021. https://www.wsj.com/articles/aging-japan -demographics-elderly-under-75-pre-old-11632490841.

Jauhar, Sandeep. "How Would You Feel about a 100-Year-Old Doctor?" *New York Times*, November 28, 2022. https://www.nytimes.com/2022/11/28/opinion /doctors-aging-competency-test.html.

"Centenarians in Japan Top 90,000 for First Time." *Japan Times*, September 16, 2022. https://www.japantimes.co.jp/tag/aging-3/?pgno=3.

Johnson, Carla K. "Next Big Wave: Radiation Drugs Track and Kill Cancer Cells." Associated Press, June 3, 2021. https://apnews.com/article/cancer-science -business-health-54e08ed1a440669a88932aba505d2e54.

Julian, Megan. "At 97, No Slowing Down This Senior Athlete." *Republican American*, August 11, 2022. Updated Link: https://archives.rep-am .com/2022/08/11/at-97-no-slowing-down-this-senior-athlete/.

Kageyama, Yuri. "World's Oldest Man, Who Said Secret Was Smiling, Dies at 112." Associated Press, February 25, 2020. https://apnews.com /article/38b32dc344e6eacd0c84044c997e51d1.

Kapcar, Jack. "Why Bernie Sanders Is so Popular with Young Voters." *Michigan Daily*, November 12, 2022. https://www.michigandaily.com/ opinion/why-bernie-sanders-is-so-popular-with-young-voters-an -account-of-his-campus-visit/.

King, Colbert. "Mr. President, as a Fellow Octogenarian, I Welcome You to the Club." *Washington Post*, November 18, 2022. https://www.washingtonpost .com/opinions/2022/11/18/biden-birthday-octogenarian-colbert-king/.

Klassen, Thomas. "70-Plus Seems the New 50 for Male Politicians, but They're Threatening the World Order." *The Conversation*, November 9, 2022. https:// theconversation.com/70-plus-seems-the-new-50-for-male-politicians -but-theyre-threatening-the-world-order-194098.

Klassen, Thomas. "Joe Biden's Win Shows the Clout of Senior Citizens in America." *The Conversation*, November 9, 2020. https://theconversation.com /joe-bidens-win-shows-the-clout-of-senior-citizens-in-america-149687.

Kolata, Gina. "A Promising Trial Targets a Genetic Risk for Alzheimer's." *New York Times*, December 2, 2022. https://www.nytimes.com/2022/12/02/health /alzheimers-apoe4-gene-therapy.html?smid=em-share.

Kole, Bill. "Kevorkian Patients: Suicide Duo's Last Words." Associated Press, October 29, 1991.

Kole, William J. "At 120 Years and 238 Days, She's World's Oldest Living Person." Associated Press, October 17, 1995.

Kole, William J. "Venerable but Vulnerable: Centenarians Hit Hard by Virus." Associated Press, May 7, 2020. https://apnews.com/article /health-us-news-ap-top-news-elderly-welfare-virus-outbreak -2a7f8b5107b6dbd93fd811c08ba15d13.

Krein, Julius. "It's Time to Depose America's Gerontocracy." *New York Post*, June 26, 2020. https://nypost.com/2020/06/26/its-time-to-depose -americas-gerontocracy/.

Levinson-King, Robin. "Canada: Why the Country Wants to Bring in 1.5m Immigrants by 2025." BBC, November 22, 2022. https://www.bbc.com/news /world-us-canada-63643912.

Lightsey, David. "National Geographic's Blue Zone Philosophy: Science or Common Sense?" *American Council on Science and Health*, January 25, 2022. https://www.acsh.org/news/2022/01/25/national-geographics-blue-zone -philosophy-science-or-common-sense-16078.

MacQuarrie, Brian. "At 108 Years Old, Cape Cod Woman Starts Fund-Raiser to Allow Her to Keep Living at Home." *Boston Globe*, July 2, 2021. https:// www.bostonglobe.com/2021/07/02/metro/108-years-old-cape-cod-woman -starts-fund-raiser-allow-her-keep-living-home/.

McFadden, Robert D. "Carmen Herrera: Carmen Herrera, Cuban-Born Artist Who Won Fame at 89, Dies at 106." *New York Times*, Feb. 13, 2022. https://www .nytimes.com/2022/02/13/arts/design/carmen-herrera-dead.html.

Miller, Alex. "Poetic Friendship: At 100 and 101, a Bond Formed through Verse." *Bozeman Daily Chronicle*, November 5, 2022. https://www .bozemandailychronicle.com/news/poetic-friendship-at-100-and-101 -a-bond-formed-through-verse/article_4b21a1c2-5c66-11ed-a29d -0fa3bc6498a4.html.

Min-sik, Yoon. "Does Korea Need a Loneliness Minister?" *Korea Herald*, August 30, 2022. https://www.koreaherald.com/view.php?ud =20220830000713.

Minutaglio, Rose. "California Man Cares for Ailing 89-Year-Old Neighbor and Best Friend in Her Final Days: 'Kindness Heals.'" *People*, January 24, 2017. https://people.com/human-interest/california-man-cares-ailing-89-year-old-neighbor-final-days/.

Moffic, H. Steven. "Aging, Ageism, and the Attitude of Youth." *Psychiatric Times*, May 9, 2022. https://www.psychiatrictimes.com/view/aging-ageism-and-the-attitude-of-youth.

Most, Doug. "Why Do Some People Live to 100—And How?" *BU Today*, September 12, 2022. https://www.bu.edu/articles/2022/why-do-people-live-to-100-and-how/.

Olen, Helaine. "As Basic Health Care Grows Unaffordable, the Rich Seek Eternal Youth." *Washington Post*, February 6, 2023. https://www.washingtonpost.com/opinions/2023/02/06/american-health-care-disparity-rich/.

Oluhemnse, Ese. "Eric Adams Strikes Celebratory Tone as Ranked Choice Count Begins." *City Limits*, June 23, 2021. https://citylimits.org/2021/06/23/eric-adams-strikes-celebratory-tone-as-ranked-choice-count-begins/.

O'Mahony, Seamus. "Are We Living Too Long?" *Saturday Evening Post*, April 30, 2019. https://www.saturdayeveningpost.com/2019/04/are-we-living-too-long/.

"Bradley Cooper on His Father's Passing: 'I've Never Seen Anything the Same Since.'" Oprah.com, February 5, 2019. https://www.oprah.com/own-supersoulsessions/bradley-cooper-reveals-lady-gagas-best-advice-about-his-singing.

Paul, Pamela. "Wait, Who Did You Say Is Middle-Aged?" *New York Times*, October 16, 2022. https://www.nytimes.com/2022/10/16/opinion/middle-age-gen-x-boomer.html.

Peltier, Elian. "A French Nun Turns 117 after Knocking Down Covid-19." *New York Times*, February 10, 2021. https://www.nytimes.com/2021/02/10/world/europe/sister-andre-covid19.html.

Perrone, Matthew. "US Regulators Lay out Plan for Over-the-Counter Hearing Aids." Associated Press, October 19, 2021. https://apnews.com/article/science-business-health-0908cbc7cfc2ee95cbc507128d5688eb.

Peterson, Elizabeth. "Sizzling Longevity: World's Oldest Person Eats Bacon Daily." Live Science, October 6, 2015. https://www.livescience.com/52406-oldest-person-eats-bacon.html.

Petrequin, Samuel. "Robert Marchand, Record-Setting Centenarian Cyclist, Dies at 109." *Washington Post*, May 22, 2021. https://www.washingtonpost.com/local/obituaries/robert-marchand-dead/2021/05/22/5041bbaa-bb0f-11eb-96b9-e949d5397de9_story.html.

Petrow, Steven. "The Anxieties of Growing Old When You're LGBTQ." *Washington Post*, October 23, 2022. https://www.washingtonpost.com/health/2022/10/23/lgbtq-aging-worries/.

Pollitt, Katha. "The Democratic Party Shouldn't Be a Gerontocracy." *The Nation*, September 2, 2022. https://www.thenation.com/article/politics/democrats-gerontocracy/.

Rabin, Roni Caryn. "3DBio Therapeutics: Doctors Transplant Ear of Human Cells, Made by 3-D Printer." *New York Times*, June 2, 2022. https://www.nytimes.com/2022/06/02/health/ear-transplant-3d-printer.html.

Rich, Motoko, and Hikari Hida. "A Yale Professor Suggested Mass Suicide for Old People in Japan. What Did He Mean?" *New York Times*, February 12, 2023. https://www.nytimes.com/2023/02/12/world/asia/japan-elderly-mass-suicide.html.

Rincon, Paul. "Predators Drove Human Evolution." *BBC News*, February 19, 2006. http://news.bbc.co.uk/2/hi/science/nature/4729050.stm.

Roll, Rich. "100 Year Old: What Really Matters In Life." *Rich Roll Podcast*, August 12, 2022. https://www.youtube.com/watch?v=Pkh8fHesypQ.

Rosenblum, Mort. "Extra: Sacre Sempé." *The Mort Report*, August 13, 2022. https://www.mortreport.org/reports/sacre-sempe.

Sabbia, Lorna. "Longer Lifespans Require Secure Financial Futures." *Boston Globe*, March 7, 2022. https://www.bostonglobe.com/2022/03/07/opinion/longer-lifespans-require-secure-financial-futures/.

Salam, Erum. "Young Voters Hailed as Key to Democratic Successes in Midterms." *The Guardian*, Nov. 11, 2022. https://www.theguardian.com/us-news/2022/nov/11/young-voters-us-midterms-democratic-youth.

Schwarcz, Joe. "Who First Suggested That Milk Be Pasteurized to Make It Safer for Consumption?" McGill University, March 20, 2017. https://www.mcgill.ca/oss/article/history-science-science-everywhere-you-asked/who-first-suggested-milk-be-pasteurized-make-it-safer-consumption.

Scott, Andrew. "The Average American Would Pay $242,000 for One Extra Year of Good Health." *Future*, September 15, 2021. https://future.com/economic-case-for-curbing-aging/.

Stobbe, Mike. "US Life Expectancy in 2020 Saw Biggest Drop Since WWII." Associated Press, July 21, 2021. https://apnews.com/article/science-health-coronavirus-pandemic-fac0863b8c252d21d6f6a22a2e3eab86.

Suderman, Peter. "Dianne Feinstein and the Dangers of Gerontocracy." *Reason*, April 15, 2022. https://reason.com/2022/04/15/dianne-feinstein-and-the-dangers-of-gerontocracy/.

Sullivan, Eric. "Kieran Culkin Bares (a Lot of) His Soul." *Esquire*, March 27, 2023. https://www.esquire.com/entertainment/a43399530/kieran-culkin-succession-interview-2023/

Tatter, Grace, and Meghna Chakrabarti. "Why Science Says Your Best Years Are Yet to Come." NPR's *On Point*, April 2, 2021. https://www.wbur.org/onpoint/2021/04/02/science-older-happier-study-pandemic.

Thomas, Jack. "I Just Learned I Only Have Months to Live. This Is What I Want to Say." *Boston Globe Magazine*, July 21, 2021. https://www.bostonglobe

.com/2021/07/21/magazine/i-just-learned-i-only-have-months-live-this
-is-what-i-want-say/.

Warburg, Gerald. "Nancy Pelosi Was the Key Democratic Messenger of Her
Generation—Passing the Torch Will Empower Younger Leadership." *The
Conversation*, November 18, 2022. https://theconversation.com/nancy-pelosi
-was-the-key-democratic-messenger-of-her-generation-passing
-the-torch-will-empower-younger-leadership-194894.

Watson, Julie Wenger. "In the Wake of the Tulsa Race Massacre's Centennial,
a Communal Hip-Hop Album Emerges." NPR, May 28, 2021. https://www
.npr.org/2021/05/28/994616024/in-the-wake-of-the-tulsa-race-massacres
-centennial-a-communal-hip-hop-album-emer.

Whitney, Craig R. "Jeanne Calment, World's Elder, Dies at 122." *New York
Times*, August 5, 1997, p. B8. https://www.nytimes.com/1997/08/05/world
/jeanne-calment-world-s-elder-dies-at-122.html.

Willingham, Emily. "Humans Could Live Up to 150 Years, New Research
Suggests." *ScientificAmerican*, May 25, 2021. https://www.scientificamerican
.com/article/humans-could-live-up-to-150-years-new-research-suggests/.

Wondracz, Aidan. "Cops Arrest 100-Year-Old Woman on Her Birthday to
Cross It off Her Bucket List." *Daily Mail Australia*, August 1, 2022. https://
www.dailymail.co.uk/news/article-11132855/Ex-army-nurse-arrested
-celebrating-100th-birthday.html.

Younger, Emily. "Three Kansas Sisters Reach Century Mark, Celebrate 104,
102 and 100 Birthday." *KSNW*, December 1, 2021. https://www.ksn.com
/community/positive-connections/three-kansas-sisters-reach-century
-mark-celebrate-104-102-and-100-birthday/.

WEBSITE CONTENT

AARP. "AARP Purpose Awards." Aug. 16, 2022. https://www.aarp.org
/about-aarp/purpose-prize/winners/info-2022/imani-woody.html.
"Giving Back to My AAPI Community Through Service." June 10, 2022.
https://www.aarp.org/experience-corps/our-stories/experience-corps
-volunteer-story-linda-fong/. "Life Is Good, Especially for Older Americans."
June 2022. https://www.aarp.org/research/topics/life/info-2022
/second-half-life-desires-concerns.html. "8 in 10 Nursing Home Residents
Given Psychiatric Drugs, Report Finds." Nov. 22, 2022. https://www.aarp.org
/caregiving/health/info-2022/psychotropic-medication-nursing-homes.html.

Aging Study of Catholic Order Members. https://www.cloisterstudy.eu/ASCOM/.

Alzheimer's Association. "Speed of Processing Training Results in Lower Risk
of Dementia." https://doi.org/10.1016%2Fj.trci.2017.09.002.

Alzheimer's Society. "The 10 Warning Signs of Dementia." 2022. https://
alzheimer.ca/en/about-dementia/do-i-have-dementia/10-warning
-signs-dementia.

American Cancer Society. "Cancer Statistics, 2023." https://doi.org/10.3322 /caac.21763.

Blue Zones.com. "Groundbreaking Blue Zones Project Expands to Canada." https://www.bluezones.com/news/groundbreaking-blue -zones-project-expands-to-canada/.

Centers for Disease Control and Prevention. "History of Smallpox." https:// www.cdc.gov/smallpox/history/history.html. "History of Drinking Water Treatment." https://www.cdc.gov/healthywater/drinking/history.html. "Chronic Disease among African American Families: A Systematic Scoping Review." http://dx.doi.org/10.5888/pcd17.190431. "Down Syndrome and Increased Risk for Alzheimer's." https://www.cdc.gov/aging/publications /features/down-syndrome-alzheimers-risk.html. "Senior Drug and Alcohol Deaths: Drug Overdose Deaths in Adults Aged 65 and Over: United States, 2000–2020. https://www.cdc.gov/nchs/products/databriefs/db455.htm.

Changing the Narrative. "Anti-ageist Birthday Card Project." https:// changingthenarrativeco.org/anti-ageist-birthday-cards/.

Diary Collection History, Congregational Library & Archives. "Ebenezer Storer." https://congregationallibrary.softlinkliberty.net/liberty/opac/ search.do?queryTerm=%22ebenezer%20storer%20diary%2C%201749 -1764.%22&mode=BASIC&=undefined&modeRadio=KEYWORD &operator=AND&timeScale=ANY_TIME&limit=All&resourceCollection =All&activeMenuItem=false.

Fight Aging. "Immune Aging Clock Identifies CXCL9 as a Target to Suppress Age-Related Inflammation." https://www.fightaging.org/archives/2021/07 /immune-aging-clock-identifies-cxcl9-as-a-target-to-suppress-age -related-inflammation/.

Guinness World Records. "I Truly Love What I Do: World's Oldest Doctor Still Working at 100." Oct. 13, 2022. https://www.guinnessworldrecords .com/news/2022/10/i-truly-love-what-i-do-worlds-oldest-doctor-still -working-at-100-721628.

Harvard University. "The Fight Over Inoculation During the 1721 Boston Smallpox Epidemic." https://sitn.hms.harvard.edu/flash/special -edition-on-infectious-disease/2014/the-fight-over-inoculation-during -the-1721-boston-smallpox-epidemic/.

Milken Institute. "Why Some People Have Longevity Genes and Others Don't." https://milkeninstitute.org/article/longevity-genes-why-some-people-have.

National Institute on Aging. "Social Isolation, Loneliness in Older People Pose Health Risks." https://www.nia.nih.gov/news/social-isolation-loneliness -older-people-pose-health-risks.

National Library of Medicine. "AD 1620: English Pilgrims Settle on Wampanoag Land." https://www.nlm.nih.gov/nativevoices/timeline/199.html.

National Museum of Civil War Medicine. "Mother I Wish I Was Out of This Place . . . Letters from a dying Civil War Soldier." https://www.civilwarmed

.org/mother-i-wish-i-was-out-of-this-place-letters-from-a-dying
-civil-war-soldier/.

Oxford Academic. "Infectious Diseases during the Civil War: The Triumph of
the 'Third Army.'" https://doi.org/10.1093/clind/16.4.580.

Pew Research Center. "World's Centenarian Population Projected to Grow
Eightfold by 2050." https://www.pewresearch.org/fact-tank/2016/04/21
/worlds-centenarian-population-projected-to-grow-eightfold-by-2050/.

"Living to 120 and Beyond: Americans' Views on Aging, Medical Advances
and Radical Life Extension." https://www.pewresearch.org/religion
/2013/08/06/living-to-120-and-beyond-americans-views-on-aging-medical
-advances-and-radical-life-extension/.

Population Reference Bureau. "How Many People Have Ever Lived on Earth?"
May 18, 2021. https://info.nicic.gov/ces/global/population-demographics
/how-many-people-have-ever-lived-earth.

Royal College of Physicians. "RCP Warns the UK Is Facing a Crisis in Care for
Older People." March 3, 2022. https://www.rcp.ac.uk/news-and-media
/news-and-opinion/rcp-warns-the-uk-is-facing-a-crisis-in-care-for
-older-people/.

Stanford Center on Longevity. "The New Map of Life." November 2021. https://
longevity.stanford.edu/the-new-map-of-life-initiative/.

The Carter Center. "Written Testimony of Former First Lady Rosalynn Carter
before the Senate Special Committee on Aging." May 26, 2011. https://www
.cartercenter.org/news/editorials_speeches/rosalynn-carter-committee-on
-aging-testimony.html.

UK government. "Loneliness Minister: 'It's More Important than Ever to Take
Action.'" https://www.gov.uk/government/news/loneliness-minister-its
-more-important-than-ever-to-take-action.

United Nations. "Global Report on Ageism—Executive Summary."
2021. https://www.who.int/teams/social-determinants-of-health
/demographic-change-and-healthy-ageing/combatting-ageism/global
-report-on-ageism.

United Nations Human Rights Council. "Older Persons Deprived of Liberty."
2022. https://awarenessweek.ipa-online.org/UserFiles/G2244700l.pdf.

US Census Bureau. "Demographic Turning Points for the United States:
Population Projections for 2020 to 2060." March 2018/revised February 2020.
https://www.census.gov/content/dam/Census/library/publications/2020
/demo/p25-1144.pdf.

Walton Family Foundation. "New Report Reveals What Issues
Motivate Gen Z and Their Future Priorities." 2023. https://www
.waltonfamilyfoundation.org/new-report-reveals-what-issues-motivate
-gen-z-and-their-future-priorities.

World Cancer Research Fund. "Worldwide Cancer Data." 2022. https://www
.wcrf.org/cancer-trends/worldwide-cancer-data/.

World Health Organization. "Ageism Is a Global Challenge." 2021. https://www
.who.int/news/item/18-03-2021-ageism-is-a-global-challenge-un.

World Population Review. "Life Expectancy by Country." https://
worldpopulationreview.com/country-rankings/life-expectancy-by-country.

Yale Medicine. "Genetic Sequencing in Heart Disease Patients Can Benefit
Families." https://www.yalemedicine.org/news/genetic-sequencing
-heart-disease-benefits.

AUTHOR INTERVIEWS

Bampoe, Vida. October 19, 2022.

Basting, Anne. October 18, 2022.

Beard, John. October 13, 2022.

Evan, Mary Anne. October 19, 2022.

Goodall, Dr. Jane. October 6, 2021.

Kole, Marie "Nadine." June 26, 2022.

Lee, Jongseong. December 11, 2022.

McCrae-Owoye, Wendy. October 13, 2022.

McKibben, Bill. December 21, 2022.

Regnante, Dr. Richard. June 30, 2021.

Perls, Dr. Thomas. August 4, 2022.

Picard, Dr. Martin. October 25, 2022.

Senhouse, Herlda. September 9, 2022.

NOTES

CHAPTER ONE: A WRINKLE IN TIME

6. "Her last . . . all of us.'": AP, "Calment." **6.** "He died . . . there himself.": NYT, "120-Year Lease." **8.** "She was . . . death and the journalists.": Kole, "Oldest Living Person." **10.** "Just four . . . US history.": Census Bureau. **12.** "Little wonder . . . two decades.": Japan Times, "Centenarians." **12.** "Half of . . . decades past.": Inada, "Pre-Old." **13.** "But she. . . 119th birthday.": Peltier, "117." **16.** "All I want is to die.": Bacon, "Indonesian." **17.** "He has yet to do so." Robine et al., "Calment." **17.** "What's most astonishing . . . ever lived to 122.": Population Reference Bureau, "How many?" **18.** "One, in Japanese . . . made death wait.": AP, "tribute." **18.** "We should not . . . living longer lives.": Olshansky, "Healthspan." **20.** Farrell, "Who'll Pay?" **20.** Elmer, "Solutions." **21.** "Systemic injustice . . . marginalized communities.": Geronimus, "Racist conditions." **21.** "In its 2021. . . target of ageism.": UN, "Ageism." **21.** Cassandra Devine: Buckley, *Boomsday.* **22.** "Consider Yusuke . . . with Boomers.": Rich, "Yale professor." **22.** Klassen, senior clout. **23.** Goodall, author interview. **26.** "Good health . . . not dread them.": AARP, "Stereotypes."

CHAPTER TWO: HOW SCIENCE LENGTHENS OUR LIVES

30. "They were smaller . . . stalking us.": Rincon, "evolution." **32.** "O Almighty God . . . distress & calamity.": Storer, diary entries. **33.** "Three years earlier . . . ravaged the tribe: National Library of Medicine, "Pilgrims." **33.** "Skulls and bones . . . a very sad spectacle to behold.": Bradford, *Of Plimoth Plantation.* **34.** "Rashes and scars . . . longer than that.": CDC, smallpox. **35.** "It didn't explode . . . pox to you.": Harvard, "inoculation." **36.** "Using the . . . dairy products.": Schwarcz, pasteurization. **37.** "Typhoid, diarrhea . . . laid their eggs.": National Library of Medicine, "infectious diseases." **37.** "Two years . . . food or water.": National Museum of Civil War Medicine, "Letters." **37.** "The Centers . . . plunged dramatically.": CDC, drinking water. **43.** "To be sure . . . among Blacks.": Stobbe, "life expectancy." **43.** "By 2050 . . . globally.": Pew, 2050. **44.** Regnante, author interview. **44.** "Scientists at . . . twenty others.": Yale, "genetic sequencing." **45**. "CRISPR technology . . . cholesterol levels.": Hamzelou, "Next up for CRISPR." **45**. "At least . . . treatment option.": Kim et al., "gene therapy." **45**. "This is a cure . . . running half-marathons.": Melenhorst et al., remissions. **46**. "Experts believe . . . hard to reach.": Johnson, radiation drugs. **46**. "It's an imperfect vaccine . . .": Greshko, malaria vaccine. **47**. "Provocative new research . . .": Willingham, "150 years." **47**. "But then . . . the current limit.": Milholland and Vijg, lifespan limits. **47**. Olshansky and Carnes, "Inconvenient Truths." **49**. "In a study . . . rodents' eyes.": Lu et al., "Reprogramming." **49**. "Researchers in . . . human aging.": Katsimpardi et al., "Vascular." **50**. "Davis points . . . the rich." Davis, "Consider the Ethics." **51**. "His theory . . . life-wrecking stress.": CBC, "Living next to water." **52**. "Will we go out with a grin . . .": Kageyama, "World's oldest man." **53**. "On the flip side . . . in the Sahara.": Xu et al., "Future."

CHAPTER THREE: THE LUCK OF THE (DNA) DRAW

55. "Bacon makes everything better.": Peterson, "Sizzling longevity." **56**. Perls, author interview. **58**. "Barzilai, who . . . move fast.": Milken Institute, "longevity genes." **60**. "Adhering to . . .": Ding et al. **63**. Anderson, Springsteen. **63**. Sullivan, Kieran Culkin interview. "Physical activity." **66**. Lipka, Pew study of Adventists. **66**. Ellison, McSweeney's satire. **67**. "Children of people 100 or older . . .": Inglés et al., "genetic footprint." **67**. Perls, author interview. **69**. "More than . . . colorectal cancer.": World Cancer Research Fund, data. **70**. "Not that . . . the vaccine.": American Cancer Society, statistics. **70**. "In the future . . . huffing and puffing.": Stanford, "The New Map of Life." **71**. Perls, author interview. **73**. "UCLA researcher . . . has aged.": Drew, epigenetic clocks. **73**. "Ever mindful . . . our subjects.'": Wu et al., gut microbiome. **75**. "We have one outlier . . .": Fight Aging, inflammation. **76**. Perls, author interview. **77**. "For families . . . historical treasure.": Kole, COVID's toll on centenarians.

CHAPTER FOUR: THE UNBEARABLE WHITENESS OF BEING A CENTENARIAN

81. "Accelerated biological aging . . . chronic conditions.": Geronimus et al., "Accelerated biological aging." **81**. "Figures from . . . high blood pressure.": CDC, "Figures from . . . high blood pressure. **81**. Smedley, National Press Foundation. **82**. Schwandt et al., life expectancy gap between races. **82**. Senhouse, author interview. **88**. "Basically Blacks . . . white counterparts.": Preston, Black mortality. **88**. Perls, author interview. **89**. "I found it . . . Robert Douglas Young.": Young, "Myth or Reality?" **89**. McCrae-Owoye, author interview. **90**. "Little wonder . . . our lifespans.": Hathaway, "Stress." **91**. Truesdale, author interview. **92**. Picard, author interview. **93**. Banerjee and Duflo: Poverty. **93**. "The story . . . Hailstork says.": Watson, "Tulsa." **95**. Truesdale, author interview. **96**. Case and Deaton, lifespan and degrees. **98**. Daniel, healthy food. **101**. "Health

disparities . . . illness or health.": Alsan, December 7, 2021: https://www
.youtube.com/watch?v=Nbud-rqQAso. **101.** Banerjee and Duflo, poverty.

CHAPTER FIVE: GROWING OLD IN A YOUTH-OBSESSED, AGEIST SOCIETY

104. "After *The Globe and Mail* . . . discrimination ensued.": Doolittle, LaFlamme.
105. Sonni Efron, Debra Whitman, National Press Foundation, September 18,
2022. **105.** Alvarez, Goodall in Denver. **107.** "For older . . . older people." WHO,
"Ageism." **107.** William Beach: National Press Foundation, September 19,
2022. **109.** "After taking older . . . elders like trash.": Horowitz, Pope Francis.
110. "Henry's only sin . . . tap ran dry.": Berkman and Truesdale, *Overtime*, 188.
110. Beth Truesdale, Ruth Finkelstein, Raymond Peeler, Bill Rivera: National
Press Foundation, September 19, 2022. **112.** Peter Gosselin: National Press
Foundation, September 19, 2022. **113.** Paul Irving: National Press Foundation,
September 20, 2022. **114.** "Few other . . . in nursing homes.": UN Human
Rights Council, liberty. **114.** Robyn Stone: Columbia University AgeBoom
Academy, October 21, 2022. **115.** Farrell et al., racism and ageism in health
care. **115.** Paul, middle age. **116.** Karon Phillips: National Press Foundation,
September 20, 2022. **116.** Gary Officer: National Press Foundation, September
20, 2022. **117.** "I've done it all my life . . .": Virginia Oliver, *TODAY*, August 13, 2022:
https://www.today.com/video/maine-s-102-year-old-lobster-lady-shows-no
-sign-of-slowing-down-146092613865. **117.** Cox, Joe Smith. **117.** McFadden,
Carmen Herrera. **117.** AP, Dagny Carlsson. **119.** Shatner: *Boldly Go*. **119.** AP,
Angela Lansbury. **120.** Changing the Narrative, ageist birthday cards. **120.**
Martha Boudreau: National Press Foundation, September 20, 2022. **122.** "I don't
get . . . *New York Times*." Hikari and Yoon, baby workers. **123.** Derenda Schubert:
Columbia University's AgeBoom Academy, October 21, 2022. **123.** Moffic, ageism.
124. Linda Fried: Columbia University's AgeBoom Academy, October 21, 2022.
125. Prengaman, September 22, 2022: https://www.youtube.com/watch?v=T-
3fKl_ZC14s. **126.** Becca Levy on loneliness: Columbia University AgeBoom
Academy, May 3, 2021: https://www.youtube.com/watch?v=EzZQUzBvT5o.

CHAPTER SIX: SILVER WITHOUT THE LINING

130. "Yet they . . . by 2100.": Pearce and Raftery, human life span by 2100.
131. Pyrkov et al., life span limit. **131.** "And a study . . . 138 years.": Podolskiy et
al., "Landscape of longevity." **132.** Higgs and Gilleard, living to 100. **132.** Rabin,
3D ear. **133.** Pew, living to 120. **133.** Davis, ethics. **134.** Olen, going without
health care. **134.** Pijnenburg and Leget, life extension. **134.** Gutin and Hummer,
inequality. **134.** Thomas, months to live. **135.** NIA, Steve Cole. **136.** Holt-Lunstad
et al., loneliness. **136.** Janine Simmons: Social Isolation and Loneliness Q&A,
NIH, March 10, 2021: https://www.youtube.com/watch?v=WBJclABlg_U.
137. Ribeiro et al., anxiety in centenarians. **137.** Brandts et al., Amsterdam

study. **136.** Holt-Lunstad et al., loneliness and social isolation. **137.** NIA, Lisbeth Nielsen **138.** Jopp et al., vulnerability and resilience. **138.** Leitch et al., New Zealand study. **140.** UK government: Baroness Diana Barran. **140.** Min-sik, Noh Woong-rae. **140.** Elmer, isolation. **142.** Kole, author interview. **144.** Basting, author interview. **145.** Foster, robots. **147.** Derenda Schubert: Columbia University's AgeBoom Academy, October 21, 2022. **148.** Tatter and Chakrabarti, Dr. Laura Carstensen **149.** Perls, author interview. **150.** Petrow, LGBTQ. **150.** AARP, Imani Woody. **151.** Dr. Justin Golub: Columbia University AgeBoom Academy, 2021. **151.** Perrone, hearing aids. **151.** Graham, is longer happier? **151.** Kole, Kevorkian.

CHAPTER SEVEN: TRIPLE-DIGIT BODIES; DOUBLE-DIGIT MINDS

155. "Doctors say . . . risk of stroke.": Fishman, "Developing dementia." **155.** Rogalski, super-aging. **157.** Beker et al., centenarian cognitive function. **157.** Perls, author interview. **158.** Quiroz et al., Alzheimer's in Latinx population. **158.** Wang et al., COVID-19 and Alzheimer's. **159:** Costumero et al., Australian research. **159.** Andersen, resistance and resilience. **159.** Perls, author interview. **160.** Vacante et al., University of Catania study. **160.** Gilbert, brain age. **161.** AP, Virginia McLaurin. **161.** Earl Mallinger: ABC. **163.** "Most of us . . . with others." Alzheimer's Society, "10 warning signs." **163.** Greco, "Goodbye." **164.** Chappell, Aaron Kesselheim. **166.** CDC, Down syndrome. **166.** Cagan et al., mutation and lifespan. **166.** "In many . . . inconclusive results.": Kolata, "A Promising Trial." **167.** Palmioli et al., University of Milan hops study. **167.** Fukuda et al., Japanese hops study. **167.** Holland et al., flavonols. **167.** Zhu et al., British study. **167.** Su et al., Chinese study. **167.** TODAY, Laura D. Baker study. **169.** Pillai et al., Bronx study. **169.** Staff et al., Scotland study. **169.** "But a landmark . . . the training." Alzheimer's Association, "Processing training." **169.** Hilliard, Elly Pollan. **171.** Breznican, Chris Hemsworth. **172.** Guinness, Dr. Howard Tucker. **172.** Jauhar, NYT essay. **172.** Tucker, letter to *NYT*, January 17, 2023. **173.** Den Dunnen et al., Hendrikje van Andel-Schipper.

CHAPTER EIGHT: EXCEPTIONALLY OLD, WITH EXTREME INFLUENCE

179. Oluhemnse, Eric Adams speech. **179.** King, aging essay. **180.** Abelson, ageism. **181.** Suderman, Dianne Feinstein. **181.** Pollitt, gerontocracy. **183.** Atella and Carbonari, European study. **184:** Klassen, aging politicians. **184:** Warburg, Pelosi. **184.** Klassen, Biden. **186.** Cristina Martin Firvida: National Press Foundation, September 19, 2022. **186:** Truesdale, author interview. **187.** Salam, Cristina Tzintzún Ramírez. **188.** Della Volpe, NYT essay. **188.** Walton Family Foundation, Gen Z survey. **189.** "If other . . . student journalist." Kapcar, "Bernie Sanders." **190.** McKibben on *PBS Newshour*, December 6, 2022: https://www.pbs.org/video/mckibben-bbs-1670368284/. **192.** Krein, America's gerontocracy. **192.** Rosenblum, Sempé. **193.** Epstein and Medina, David Axelrod. **193.** Carey,

S. Jay Olshansky. **195**. Paul Irving: National Press Foundation, September 20, 2022. **196**. William Beach, National Press Foundation, September 19, 2022. **197**. Coughlin, *The Longevity Economy.* **198**. AP, Judge Wesley Brown. **199**: Daley, Iris Apfel. **200**. AARP, Linda Fong. **201**. Beard, Columbia University's AgeBoom Academy, October 13, 2022. **201**. Beard, author interview.

CHAPTER NINE: WHO WILL CARE FOR US? AND WHO WILL PAY?

205. MacQuarrie, Juliet Bernstein. **206**. RCP, Britain's doctor shortage. **206**. Farrell, who pays? **207**. Caregiver support ratio: AARP Public Policy Institute, August 2013. **207**. Debra Whitman: National Press Foundation, September 18, 2022. **208**. Jason Resendez: Columbia University's AgeBoom Academy, October 14, 2022. **208**. Catherine Collinson, John Schall, Yulya Truskinovsky: Columbia University's AgeBoom Academy, October 2022. **209**. Beard, author interview. **210**. Lee, author interview. **211**. Linda Fried, Columbia University's AgeBoom Academy, October 21, 2022. **211**. Stanford, "The New Map of Life." **211**. The Carter Center, Rosalynn Carter. **212**. Sheria Robinson-Lane, Susan Reinhard, John Schall: Columbia University's AgeBoom Academy, October 2022. **213**. Paul Irving, National Press Foundation, September 20, 2022. **213**. Oprah.com, Bradley Cooper. **213**. Greg Link, Columbia University, December 1, 2022. **214**. Joseph Fuller: Columbia University's AgeBoom Academy, October 20, 2022. **215**. Jennifer Wolff: Columbia University's AgeBoom Academy, October 14, 2022. **215**. Ruth Finkelstein: National Press Foundation, September 20, 2022. **216**. David Grabowski, Robert Espinoza: Columbia University's AgeBoom Academy, October 2022. **217**. Chapman et al., personal care aides. **217**. Fraser and Penzenstadler, *USA Today* nursing home investigation. **217**. AARP, "chemical straitjackets." **218**. Schafer et al., living alone. **218**. Robyn Stone: Columbia University's AgeBoom Academy, October 21, 2022. **220**. Levinson-King, Canada immigration. **220**. Bampoe and Evan: Columbia AgeBoom Academy and author interviews. **222**. Debra Whitman: National Press Foundation, September 18, 2022. **223**. David John: National Press Foundation, September 20, 2022. **224**. Sabbia, financial futures. **224**. Jean Accius: National Press Foundation, September 20, 2022. **225**. Siavash Radpour: National Press Foundation, September 20, 2022. **225**. Truesdale, author interview. **226**. RAND, China military spending. **226**. Dong, China's elder rights law. **226**. Minutaglio, Chris Salvatore and Norma Cook. **227**. Salvatore Instagram post, February 15, 2017: https://www.instagram.com/accounts/login/?next=%2Fp%2FBQjFlZeDfBY%2F&source=desktop_nav. **227**. Van Dyke: *Keep Moving.*

CHAPTER TEN: BELIEF, POSITIVITY, AND THE TRUTH ABOUT "BLUE ZONES"

230. Whitney, Jean-Marie Robine. **232**. Lewina et al., BU optimism study. **232**. Koga et al., optimism in aging women. **232**. Almeida et al., Penn State

University study. **232**. AARP, survey with NatGeo. **233**. Basting, author interview. **233**. CDC, senior drug and alcohol deaths. **233**. Levy et al., Yale study of positivity. **234**. Julian, Madeline Smith. **234**. Wondracz, Jean Bicketon. **235**. Wallace et al., Ohio State University study. **235**. Li et al., Harvard nurses study. **236**. Wong et al., Portuguese study. **236**. Younger, Kansas centenarian sisters. **236**. Bryner, Richard Overton. **237**. Goodall, author interview. **241**. Newman, Blue Zones. **241**. Lightsey, Blue Zone philosophy. **242**. Kreouzi et al., University of Nicosia study. **242**. ASCOM, Luy study of monks and nuns. **243**. BlueZones.Com, projects in Canada and Coachella. **243**. Chu, Ephraim Engleman. **244**. Petrequin, Robert Marchand. **244**. Araújo et al., Portugal study. **245**. AP, Mimi Reinhard. **245**. Most, Perls on BU podcast. **245**. Profil, Daniela Jopp. **246**. Roll, Mike Fremont. **246**. McKibben, author interview. **247**. Jia and Lubetkin, selection bias in marriage research. **248**. Miller, Bob Yaw and Gloria Hansard. **250**. World Population Review, Africa life expectancy. **250**. Emanuel, dying at 75. **251**. Scott, cost of extra life. **251**. O'Mahony, *Saturday Evening Post* essay. **255**. Butler, gerontocracy. **256**. Oliver, "The Summer Day," *House of Light*.

INDEX

ABOUT THE AUTHOR

WILLIAM J. KOLE, recently retired as the New England news editor for the Associated Press, is a veteran journalist and former foreign correspondent who has reported from North America, Europe, Africa, and the Middle East. The grandson of a woman who lived to just shy of 104, Kole has been writing about extreme longevity since the 1990s, when he was based in Paris and told the world the extraordinary story of Jeanne Calment, who lived to 122. His many awards include one from the Society of American Business Editors & Writers for an investigation into the exploitation of undocumented immigrants by the Walmart retail chain. A 2022 fellow in aging journalism at Columbia University in New York and at the National Press Foundation in Washington, DC, he speaks English, French, Dutch, and German, and resides in Warwick, Rhode Island. This is his first book.

Printed in the United States
by Baker & Taylor Publisher Services